The Survival Guide for Kids

A Basic How to Survive and be Prepared in the Wilderness

Weise Weasel

Table of Contents

Introduction..1

Chapter 1: What to do If You Get Lost?................................3

Chapter 2: How to Signal for Help......................................9

Chapter 3: How to Find Water..17

Chapter 4: How to Build a Fire...24

Chapter 5: How to Create a Shelter....................................33

Chapter 6: How to Stay Safe From Wild Animals.............48

Chapter 7: First Aid Tips to Keep You Safe.......................65

Chapter 8: How to Deal with Bugs on the Trail................74

Chapter 9: Tips About Foraging for Food..........................87

Chapter 10: Learning How to Navigate...........................100

Chapter 11: Keeping Your Shelter Area Clean...................111

Chapter 12: Keeping Dry When it Rains..........................120

Chapter 13: How to Survive Extreme Weather................131

Conclusion..151

© Copyright 2018 by Weise Weasel - All rights reserved.

The follow eBook is reproduced below with the goal of providing information that is as accurate and reliable as possible. Regardless, purchasing this eBook can be seen as consent to the fact that both the publisher and the author of this book are in no way experts on the topics discussed within and that any recommendations or suggestions that are made herein are for entertainment purposes only. Professionals should be consulted as needed prior to undertaking any of the action endorsed herein.

This declaration is deemed fair and valid by both the American Bar Association and the Committee of Publishers Association and is legally binding throughout the United States.

Furthermore, the transmission, duplication or reproduction of any of the following work including specific information will be considered an illegal act irrespective of if it is done electronically or in print. This extends to creating a secondary or tertiary copy of the work or a recorded copy and is only allowed with express written consent from the Publisher. All additional right reserved.

The information in the following pages is broadly considered to be a truthful and accurate account of facts and as such any inattention, use or misuse of the information in question by the reader will render any resulting actions solely under their purview. There are no scenarios in which the publisher or the original author of this work can be in any fashion deemed liable for any hardship or damages that may befall them after undertaking information described herein.

Additionally, the information in the following pages is intended only for informational purposes and should thus be thought of as universal. As befitting its nature, it is presented without assurance regarding its prolonged validity or interim quality. Trademarks that are mentioned are done without written consent and can in no way be considered an endorsement from the trademark holder.

Introduction

The following chapters will discuss everything that you need to know in order to survive in the wilderness. Getting lost out in the wilderness can be scary. You are not sure where you are, it may be getting dark, and you want to make sure that you stay safe. With the information in this guidebook, you will learn how to take care of yourself when you do get lost out in the wilderness, and the steps that you need to make sure someone is able to find you.

This guidebook has a lot of great topics to discuss in order to keep you safe. We will talk about what to do when you first get lost, how to create a fire and a shelter to stay warm, how to find good water and purify it to keep it safe, how to signal for help, how to find your own food when you are out for a long time, and even how to protect yourself when you have extreme weather conditions going on around you. All of this comes together to provide you with a comprehensive idea of how you can behave and survive in the wilderness.

When you are ready to learn more about surviving in the wild and increasing your chances of surviving if you do happen to get lost, make sure to read through this guidebook to help you get started.

There are plenty of books on this subject on the market, thanks again for choosing this one! Every effort was made to ensure it is full of as much useful information as possible, please enjoy!

Chapter 1: What to do If You Get Lost?

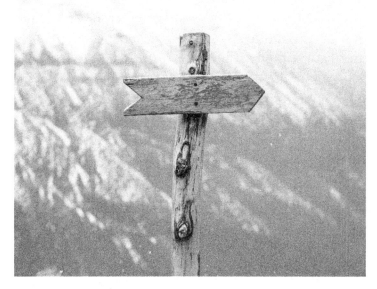

The first thing that we need to look at is what you should do if you get lost. Knowing how to react when you get lost can make it easier to follow some of the other tips that we have in this guidebook. Realizing that you are lost can be a scary feeling and sometimes other emotions will get in the way of letting you be in complete control of the situation. However, the biggest tool that you have at your disposal when it comes to survival is your brain.

So, when you first realize that you are lost, make sure to stay calm and take some deep breaths. You will survive and someone will find you; it is likely that someone will find you really soon. Your main job at this point is to stay protected and healthy until someone is able to find you. This can be easier said than done though. If you find that you are panicking a little bit, it is important to take a deep breath and just say STOP.

STOP is an acronym that you can use to take control when you are lost and your emotions are starting to take over. It stands for the following:

- **S**: This stands for Stop. This is the time that you stop your emotions right now.

Sometimes it is all about stopping what you are doing and staying in one place. The more that you move around, the harder it will be for someone to find you later on. It is a good idea to tell yourself tat it will be fine and then figure out how to stay in one place while keeping yourself safe.

- **T**: This is for think. After you have had a little bit of time to take deep breaths, it is time to start thinking. Do you know your current location? Who has an idea of where you are? What you can use around you to make things better? How many hours do you have before it gets dark? Will you need to make a shelter to stay safe? These questions will help you to determine what the next step will be for you.
- **O**: This is for observe: You should around you and observe what you can see. You can look around and see what can be used for bedding, what can be used for water, and even for a place to use to signal others.
- **P**: This is for plan. Now that you have had time to think and observe what is going on around you, it is time to decide what you would like to accomplish and in what order you would like to do them in.

The first thing that you need to worry about is your safety. So start by looking to see if you are in a safe spot. If you are high up on a hill or a mountain, or you are dealing with a thunderstorm, it is time to get down to some lower ground as soon as you can. You should always be careful about being near big trees or boulders because if there is a storm with some lightening, you should stay away from these spots as lightning is most likely to strike here.

The next thing that you should consider is whether you will need to protect yourself from bad weather and if you will need to make a fire to help stay warm. If these are things that are needed, you should make sure that they are at the top of your list. Plan where you will look in order to find the materials that are needed to build a shelter and see if you are able to find some wood for the fire. As you are collecting your firewood, bring in more than you think you will need because there is never too much of this.

You also need to take some time to look for water. It is a good idea to look or a good supply so that you stay hydrated. It is important to find a good water supply that is nearby. If you have to wander around too much to find the water, you may end up getting lost even more.

And finally, you should think of some ways that you will be able to make it easier for people to find you. A space that is nice and open will be the best because it makes it more likely that a helicopter or an airplane will be able to find you. Are you able to find a place where you can build up a signal fire? Or can you even make an X with rocks or some other material?

There is help on the way

If you do go missing, remember that it will not take too long before someone comes to look for you. The first thing that your parents will do is notify a park ranger or the police. These officials will then be able to call search and rescue in order to come find you. They are also trained to help with wilderness survival skills so will be able to help you with knot-tying, navigation, and first aid.

There are a variety of people who will be on the search and rescue team. These can include volunteers, sheriffs, deputies, and park rangers. Some will work as ground pounders who are going to travel on foot to find people who got lost, and there are also who will serve as ATV drivers and will search through trails and back roads. Other helpers will be those with search dogs, those who drive the helicopters, and more.

There are going to be a ton of people who will be out there searching for you. Your job is to stay in a place that makes it easier to be found and ensure that you are safe. There are lot of kids who are gong to do something that makes it harder for them to be rescued. They may sometimes will choose to hide from people; this could be because they were trained to not talk to strangers, or they may be worried that they will be in trouble because they wandered off and got lost. There have been cases where the searchers were right from a lost kid, but the child stayed hidden because they were worried about what would happen if the were found.

It is important to realize that this is really dangerous behavior. The search and rescue team is risking their time and lives in order to find you. It is important that you do as much as you can so that the search and rescue team is able to find you.

Chapter 2: How to Signal for Help

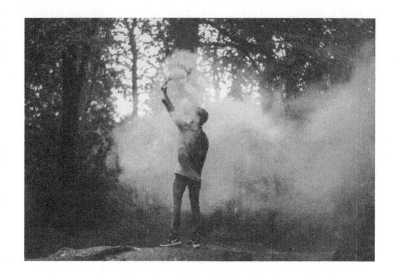

After you have taken some time to create your shelters and found a good supply of water (which we will discuss later on), it is time to signal for help so that someone else is able to find you. You know that someone is already looking for you and you may have even seen a helicopter or something else flying over and searching for you. It may be hard for them to figure out where you are though unless they are right on top of you. This is why it is so important for you to start signaling so that someone has a better chance of locating you.

To make sure that you attract the attention of the searchers, you must make sure that you stand out. There are several ways to do this, depending on your location, what the weather is like at the time, and the methods that you think the searchers are using in order to find you.

Air horns and whistles

If you get lost when it is night time, it is going to be hard for people to see you in the dark. But they may have a chance to hear you, no matter what time of day. Yelling is one place to start, but the person who is looking for you has to be relatively close in order to hear you so this is not the most effective method to use. A better idea to go with is to carry a whistle. These whistles will not take much energy on your part, they will not make you lose your voice from using them, and you will be able to make a sound that carries much further than your own voice.

There are a ton of whistles that you are able to use, and there are even some options that come off twice as loud as regular whistle and some that are good for underwater. Make sure tat whatever one you choose, you get it without the pea inside; if the pea gets wet, the whistle will not work.

You can also choose to carry a smaller air horn with you. These are good for signaling and can also be good if you need to scare off mountain lions or bears. There are some emergency air horns that are compact and will fit into your hand. These are good options that can keep you safe will signal your location, and will not take up too much space in your bag.

The signal that you should use to show that you need help is three loud noises with a break in between each of the blasts. So, if you are using the whistle or the air horn, you can do sets of three blasts, wait about a minute, and then do another set of three. Make sure to cover up your ears if you are using the air horn because these can be really loud and will hurt your ears.

Chemical light sticks and flashlight

A flashlight or a headlamp is great for signaling someone after it gets dark. You will be able to add some more attention to it by moving the light around or back and forth. You do not want to keep one of these on all night though because it will wear out the batteries.

A chemical light stick is a better option if you would like to keep the light on even while you are asleep. You will be able to get these to light up your area for most of the night without having to waste out batteries. However, these light sticks will require someone to be pretty close to you before they are able to see you. When you are ready to use these light sticks, you will bend them a little bit until you her a pop. Then shake the light stick and they will light up.

Ground signals

If you are on the ground and you would like to signal a plane or a helicopter that is overhead, you must make sure that you are out in open ground. You will be seen better when wearing a color that stands out, such as orange. Even if you are able to bring out an orange trash bag, it will increase your chances of being seen. Wave around the trash bag or choose to lie down on your back and move your legs and arms so that you appear larger and have a better chance of getting attention.

It is also possible to make a sign that appears on the ground. It is not necessary to spend time writing out a whole word; simply making a big X will do the trick. You can use rocks, wood, or anything that you see around you that is easily seen from the sky. If you are in the snow, you can even use your feet to make the X, just make sure that the letter is really big so that the pilots can see what you did from above.

Other items that may help

There are also several other survival kit items that you can bring along and use to make yourself more visible. Some of the options that you can go with will include:

- Flagging tape: Flagging tape is usually long and bright orange. You can take these and place them close together to make an X and then you will be seen from a long way away. You must hold down these strips with some rocks or dirt so that they don't end up blowing away.
- Flavored gelatin: Since the bright colors are going to show up well against white snow, one thing that you are able to do is take some cherry gelatin and scatter it over the snow to make an X that is really easy to see.
- Mylar-lined tarp: These are known as space blankets, but they are tarps that are created from a silvery material that can be good of signaling. You should fasten them down into the ground to ensure they stay in put.

Signal fires and signal mirrors

A signal fire or mirror is a good way to get the attention of a plane or a helicopter as well as those who are searching for you on the ground. A signal mirror will be a simple mirror that has a hole in the center. This hole is going to allow you to look through the mirror so that you can see what you are doing while you aim the signal. By tipping the mirror a bit n your hand, you will be able to direct a flash of sun to the rescuers, even if they are up to 50 miles away. If you are using this method and it looks like the pilot has seen you, be extra careful with this signal because you could end up blinding the pilot.

If you did not bring along a signal mirror to help you, you can also use the mirror that comes in your compass. The review mirror of your car will work well, a CD, bright piece of metal, and more.

Another option to go with is a signal fire. To start this this, you need to clear out about ten feet, making sure that all flammable material is out of the way. You can start your fire right in the middle of this area. If you see or hear someone who is trying to find you and who may notice the signal, you can add some wet leaves or fresh material on the fire. This will cause some white smoke to appear and will make your signal more noticeable.

When you are doing this, make sure that you are not using wet logs or branches. These will sometimes pop and will send out some fiery sparks to you. Never burn poison ivy or oak because the smoke is dangerous. The safest place to do this are on rocky areas or sandy areas that are near the water and are away from anything that may catch on fire. Make sure to avoid hanging branches, pine needles, and dried grass.

Walkie-talkies and cell phones

It is a good idea to carry a walkie-talkie or a cell phone with you no matter where you go. It is sometimes necessary for you to use both because there may be some places where you will not get cell service. Even if you are somewhere where you are not able to make calls, you can try to send a text message and it may go through.

Many phones now have GPS functions built into them. This is good news because even if you do not have a phone signal and don't have the ability to call someone, it is possible that your cell phone company will be able to find you. This will only work if you have this kind of feature on your phone and the phone is turned on, but it can be a way to help save you.

Chapter 3: How to Find Water

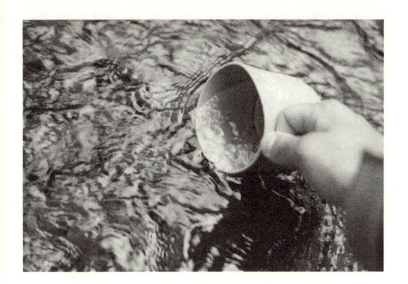

Think about the rule of three when you get lost. This rule states that you will be able to survive about three hours without shelter in extreme weather, but at most, you will only be able to survive three days without water. Water is going to be an urgent need when you are in a survival situation.

To make sure that you are healthy and hydrated, you will need to drink at least 64 to 96 ounces of water each day. if you are feeling sick, if you are out in the hot weather for a long period of time, if you are doing physical labor, or if you are exercising, it is possible that you will need a lot more water.

Whenever you decide to explore the wilderness or you would like to go on a hike, consider bringing along at least two full 32-ounce bottles of water. You can find some good plastic ones at sporting goods ad camping stores. That way, if you do get lost, you at least have some water on you. If you become lost, you should start looking for another source of fresh water before your current water supply is gone. Do not stray too far from the rescuers on this one because it makes it harder to find you. Also, remember that most lake water and river water needs to be purified, but we will talk about how to do this later.

No matter how thirsty you become while you are lost, it is not safe to drink water from the ocean, or any other source of salt water. Drinking from these water sources will simply flush out the extra water in your body to get rid of the salt, and it is basically a faster way to become hydrated.

You know that you are getting thirsty and need more water when you feel that your mouth is sticky and dry. You may have some other symptoms like dizziness, tiredness, weakness, and trouble in the stomach. If you do not have a lot of water supply left and you have not been able to find a good supply to work with, never start running around. Rest in the shade, keep your head covered and preserve your energy as much as possible.

Now that we know how important water can be to your survival in the wilderness, it is time to talk a bit more about how to find water and other water related topics.

Locating your water

The cleanest natural source of fresh water for you to drink will be springs, fast flowing streams, and snow. Then you can use ponds and lakes. And then you can move on to marshy and wet areas, outside of the ocean which you should never drink from. With some of the latter choices, you may need to purify the water before you are able to drink it.

The lower you are in elevation, the more likely it is that the water will have contaminants in it. However, it is also more likely that you will find water if you are lower in elevation.

It is important that you are able to find the right sources of water. You should try to find a spring if there is one close enough to you. This will usually be if you are higher up in elevation, but they are nice and pure and are less likely to have bad contaminants and bugs inside. Finding a good lake or a stream can work well too. It is best to reach as close to the bottom as possible with these because most experts agree that the bad stuff in lakes and streams, the stuff that can make you sick, is going to be found at the surface of these bodies of water.

You may also want to consider setting up something that will help to catch rainwater. Depending on where you are, this could at least give you something to rely on when it comes to drinking water, and this water will not need to be purified like other sources will. It does not hurt to just leave this up, even if it does not rain each day.

You may also be able to get some of your water from the plants around you. if there are some plants, especially berries, these can be safe to eat and will help to give you a little dose of water.

Purifying your water

It is going to be really hard to find water that is completely clean to drink. It most areas you will find that there are lots of tiny creatures and contaminants in the streams, lakes, and rivers that you would like to use as water sources. The water may seem clear, but if you looked at it through a microscope, you would see a lot of things that could make you sick.

While this may be enough to make you not feel like drinking the water at all, it will not take too long before your body needs more water. The good news is that there are several ways that you are able to make your water safe. The easiest method to us is going to include water purification tablets. These are made from chlorine and iodine and they do not take up that much room in your pack. You will be able to fill up a 32-ounce water bottle, drop in a tablet, shake it around, and then wait a little bit (look at the package to see if it is between one to four hours), and then you have clean water.

These tablets are very effective for cleaning out your water and making it safe to drink, but the taste will not be that great. Some people who use these iodine tablets will carry around packets of powdered vitamin C drink mix to add to the water.

Another option is to go with some water purification devices that have special filters that will help to clean the water that is in your bottles or will allow you to sip the water through a straw. There are even options that use UV lights to kill off parasites, germs, and viruses. All you will need to do with these options is to stick them inside the bottle of water and turn them on. You can pick which purification device you would like to use, but just learn how to use it before you even go out so that it doesn't become a liability.

If you are out in the wilderness and you do not have some kind of purification device on you, it is possible to boil your water to kill off the germs and tiny creatures that would make you sick. This is a method that has been around for a long time. All you need to do to make this work is to bring out a container and start a fire. Add the water to the container and let it boil for a minute. Then allow the water to cool down before you drink it.

If the only water you are able to find is in muddy water, it is possible to filter out the dirt with the help of a bandana or some clothing. You could also pour your water through some sand to help remove the mud. If you have a fire, the crushed charcoal that comes from the burned wood is good for filtering the water, and can be used to make the water taste better. Carrying some coffee filters when you hike can be a good idea to use when you need to filter out the muddy water. Even after you have used a filter to get rid of the mud from your water, you will still need to boil or purify the water to make it safe to drink.

Water is one of the most important things that you will need to do when it comes to surviving. Your body will not be able to go very long without water, and it is critical that you drink enough to stay hydrated. Starting your search for some water early on when you get lost will make it easier to survive, no matter how long it takes for the rescuers to find you.

Chapter 4: How to Build a Fire

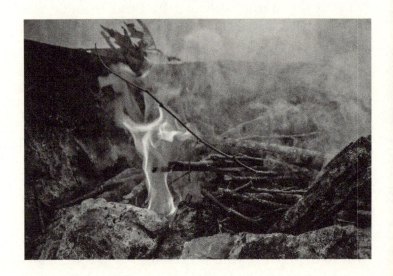

The ability to build your own fire is a good skill to learn. A campfire when you go out with friends and family can keep you safe and warm. It will help to be a signal to the rescuers who are looking for you at night. It will help to keep away those scary animals. It can also be something that is able to save your life. But if you do not know how to take care of the fire and you do not know how to use it properly, you could burn yourself, set the shelter on fire, and even start a forest fire.

To keep things simple, your fire needs fuel, heat, and air. This may seem pretty simple, but what about if you set a campfire on a rainy day? What about if you are scared and tired and it is already dark outside? It is possible to use the whole book of matches that you have just to start one fire and you are all out of luck.

This is why you need to take some time to look through this chapter. We are going to take some time to look through the steps that you need to follow in order to build up a fire and get it to serve you. There are so many benefits of using a fire, from keeping you warm to cooking to keeping animals away, but for your own safety, you need to know how to properly build up a fire that can keep you safe.

How to prepare the area for a fire

The first thing that you need to do is pick a place that is naturally fire safe. This would include places like on a sandy area or on a large rock. You must keep the fire out of the wind if you can and having a rock wall or a boulder behind it can help. Having this large rock right there will allow more of the heat to reflect back to you so you are able to stay warmer.

It is always a good idea to clear out a big area around your fire, even if you are planning on making a small fire. This will help you to avoid starting a fire that will get out of control. This means that you will need to remove pine needles grasses, and flammable leaves from the area. If possible, try to make your own fire pit by digging a hole a few inches deep where you want to place the fire. This is going to help make your fire safer and easier to start if there is a breeze. If you can't get that pit done, place some rocks around the fire to keep the flames contained.

Now, if you are in an area that has a lot of snow, you will need to take some extra steps. You will not be able to do the fire right in the snow or it will just die out with the moisture. You will need to build up a little deck of sticks or logs and then do the fire on there.

After you are ready with your fire ring or a deck or a fire pit, it is time to gather the materials that are needed for the fire. You want to get a lot of wood, much more than you think you will need if you want it to last through the night. you will need to find a combination of big logs, kindling sticks, and smaller pieces of tinder. The tinder will be what you light first to get the fire going, the kindling will be the branches and the sticks that help the fire stay strong. The tinder you pick will need to be dry and the fluffier you can find it, the better.

Types of tinder you can choose

It is a good idea to carry some tinder in your survival kit. The best types of tinder materials that you can use include pieces of fatwood, waxed paper, shredded paper, and fine steel wool. You can also use some dryer lint if you have any in your pockets with you. If you were not able to bring any tinder with you and the weather outside is wet, you should look for small parts of bark or wood, or dry grass and pine needles. If everything is wet, the best thing that you can go with is punk, or rotted wood found inside trees and has been dead for awhile.

While you are searching for the firewood that you would like to use, always search somewhere that is protected, as much as possible, from the weather. Under a large tree, or beneath some bark of a tree will help. Get at least enough to start the fire. You can always place some damp pieces near the fire to warm up before you use them as long as the fire is already going.

There are several methods that help you to build a fire, but all of them include you beginning by lighting small pieces of dry tinder. You should arrange your tinder to keep it protected from the wind, but it is not smothered. You can try making a small tepee of tinder and small sticks, or you can just let the tinder be against a log. Once the tinder has a flame with it, gently blow on the fire to add some oxygen while slowly feeding in some small kindling sticks. You will only want to do a few sticks at a time as the fire builds up. Only when you have a strong fire will you be able to add larger sticks and then logs.

Fire starting materials

Once you have gotten the tinder ready, it is time to light it. Most of the time you will be able to use a bow drill a fire plow or flint. With the flint, you will be able to create some sparks that you will use to light the fire. With the bow drills and the fire plows, you will rub two sticks so that they create the heat and friction that you need. While these methods can be fun to learn, they are not the most effective methods to use, especially if you are cold and alone in the woods.

This is why it is a good idea to bring along some fire starters in your survival kit. Waterproof matches will help you to start a fire easily no matter the weather conditions, disposable lighters can help as well. It is worth your time to bring both along so that you are prepared when you go hiking.

These are not the only things that you can use to help start a fire. There are other items that you can add into the tinder to make it easier to start the fire and getting it to really grow. Some of the other items that you can use include:

- Tortilla chips: If you hold your flame under a tortilla chip for only a few seconds, it can catch fire. The best ones to use re those that are light in color and do not have a lot of seasoning on them. you can also go with potato chips and corn chips.
- Candle wax and toilet paper: For this, you can coat individual toilet paper pieces with some melted candlewax. These won't take long to catch on fire and they last for a long time.
- Petroleum jelly on cotton balls: You can dip some cotton balls into Vaseline and get them to catch on fire right away. These will burn strong with a big flame, for at least long enough that you can light the tinder.
- Fire paste: This is sold in tubes and you simply squeeze it onto the wood before lighting it. This will ignite the log right away.
- Fuel tablets: You will have your choice of fuel tablets that you can work with and they burn well. This is a good option to work with if you need enough heat to cook your food.
- Magnesium block scrapings: These will be sold in blocks with a flint edge that helps create sparks. Using your knife, you will shav a bit of the flakes onto the tinder and it will start a fire.

If you get lost in the wilderness and you did not bring any materials to help you start a fire, then it is time to look around you to see which items you are able to use as substitutes. Is there some lint in your pocket or some tissues? Do you have some wrappers from your food or a corner of a map to use? You may have to be creative to ensure that you can stay warm and safe when starting your own fire.

Keep warm and safe

To stay warm with your fire at night, you simply need to heat up a few rocks next to your fire and then place these inside your shelter. These are going to be really hot so handle them with care so you do not get burnt. These will need about an hour to cool down, and even then you should place something on your hands to carry these.

With this rock, you should not place it into or near the fire if the rock has been sitting in water or if there are small cracks or pockets that are able to trap water. These pockets of air can be dangerous because they will make the rock explode suddenly when you heat it up too much. You should be careful when choosing your rocks to heat up because it is possible that snakes, scorpions and other animals may be under them.

When you are ready to leave your camp the next day, make sure that you extinguish your fire. This is true whether you plan to come back that day or you are moving on for good. If you have enough supply, pour some water on the fire and then stir it with a stick to make sure it is out. If you do not have water, cover the fire with a good layer of sand or dirt. Always double and triple check that the fire is gone before you head out. there are many times that a brush fire or a forest fire will start because campfires are not properly taken care of. Always treat the fire with the utmost respect and do not let your carelessness or your being in a hurry cause some unneeded danger.

Chapter 5: How to Create a Shelter

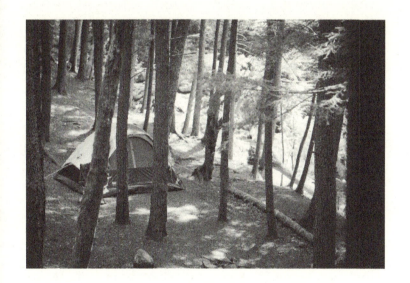

Another thing that you are going to need to focus on is building a shelter. If you are lost and working on your survival plan, it is important to keep in mind the rule of three. The rule of three is gong to be that you are only gong to be able to live about three weeks without food, three days without water, but only three hours without having a good shelter if the weather is really extreme. This means that you need to get a shelter up and running as soon as you can.

It is common that most people will get lost later in the afternoon, which means that you will need to work fast in order to get that shelter ready to go as soon as possible. Even if you are just camping or going out on an adventure, rather than being lost, it is still important that finding a shelter is one of the first things that you do.

There are a lot of benefits that come with creating a shelter. It is good at keeping you warm when the weather is warm and cool when it is hot. It will protect you from bad weather conditions, such as snow and rain. And it makes it easier to fall asleep. You will find that there are many types of shelters that you are able to choose and often it will depend on the tools that you can find and the materials that are close to you. Let's take a look at some of the things that you should consider when it comes to building your shelter.

Choose the right location

The first thing that you should consider is where you should build your shelter. If you are worried about the cold, it is a good idea to pick a spot that is about halfway up the hill and somewhere that is sunny. This is going to be the warmest spot for you. If you are not able to find a hill, it is a good idea to camp near a big rock that is in the sun most of the day.

On the other hand, if you are looking to keep out of the heat, you should use a place that is close to the water. This could help to keep the temperature down by ten degrees or so compared to being up on a hill. If you are by the water, remember that there are going to be a lot of company there. You will have to worry about flies, mosquitos, and bees. Also, it is important to be aware that there are some rivers and streams will raise a few feet overnight so you must keep your shelter a bit away.

If you happen to get lost in the desert, you should never put your shelter near a canyon or a dry riverbed. These areas can end up being right in the path of a flash flood without much warning. This can make it really unsafe to stay there.

It is a good idea to pick out a location that is close to a trail because this makes it easier for hikers and rescuers are able to find you easier. Of course, this dos not mean that your shelter should be right on the trail or right next to it. There are a lot of wild animals, such as coyotes, bars, bobcats, mountain lions, skunks, and deer you will wonder on these trails at night and you probably do not want to deal with these visitors while you are sleeping.

At this point, you may be curious to find out how you will be able to pick a safe spot. First, you should make sure that you are protected if there are any strong winds that come up. You will want to make sure that there are no big trees around so that the dead branches that might fall on you. You should also check out to see if any trees near you are struck by lightening. If you see these, that means that you are in a danger zone for lightning so you should avoid these places. If you are worried about lightning, it is best to stay away from lone trees, open spaces, high rocks, and mountaintops.

In addition, it is a good idea to pick out a spot that is not claimed by small biting craters, such as ants and ticks. You can also kick away leaves and needles to see if there are any problems like spiderwebs or scorpion holes that will make you uncomfortable while you are sleeping.

And finally, you should make sure that there are plenty of materials nearby to help you to build a shelter. If you find that there is a spot that will not provide you with enough building material, it is time to move to a different spot.

A good activity that you can do is the next time that you go out on a hike or a walk, take a look around you and try to figure out where you would be able to build a shelter and if there are plenty of items around for you to use as a shelter. Practicing this a few times will make it easier if you are dealing with being lost for real.

So, how long is it going to take in order to build up your own shelter> You will find that you will need at least an our and a half to find all the materials that you need to build this shelter. Of course, you do want to get the materials and the shelter built before it gets dark. How are you able to tell when the sun is going to set? You are able to do this by using your hand.

To do this, just hold your arm straight out with the palm facing you and the fingers together. Line up the pinky so that it is even with the horizon. The space that is taken up by the four fingers is going to be one hour and the space of one finer will be 15 minutes. You can then count how many hands and fingers there are until the sun reaches the horizon and that will tell you how long it will be until sunset.

The rules to build a shelter.

Once you have been able to choose the right site for your shelter, the next step that you should take is to plan how much room you will need in order to create the shelter. It is important to do this before you make the walls of your shelter. You do not want to spend all that time creating a good shelter and then find out that it is so small that you are not able to fit inside of it. Your shelter does not need to be huge, but it needs to be large enough so that you are able to lie down inside of it. When it comes to staying warm, the smaller the better with the shelter because it will help to trap in some more of your body heat compared to a large shelter.

It is also important that you never sleep on the bare ground, especially in cold weather. This cold ground is going to take all the body heat out of you.

If you do not have anything with you to use as your bedding it is possible to use some natural bedding that you make out of pine cones, pine boughs, pine needles, and so on. If you are able to be around some soft bedding materials, you are in luck. The thicker that you are able to make the bedding, the warmer you will be. It is best to make a bed that is at least twice as thick as you think that you will need to help you stay warm and be comfortable.

Learning the right knots

To make it easier to build a good shelter, it is important that you know how to tie some knots. Although, there are hundreds of knots, but it is only important that you learn how to work with a few of them. Basic knots, like the bowline, will help you to tie together the central support of the shelter to a tree or when you need to hang up the food stash so that the bears are not able to get to it. These are simple to learn how to work with and can be untied really quickly so that you have the ability to reuse that rope.

The best way for you to learn how to work with a knot is to watch how others do them and then practice with your own rope. Some of the most common knots that you will work with include:

- Bowline: This is considered the most basic knot. It is used to attach a single rope over to something like a tree. It is easy to tie and untie, except when the rope will be stretched taut with some kind of weight. In order to tie a bowline, you should make a small loop in the rope. Then you are able to bring the end of the rope through the loop, around the rope, and back down into the loop and pull it tight.
- Clove hitch: This is used to tie something like a tarp to a pole. It is useful because you are able to adjust the rope length as you tie it, which will make it easier to tie a tarp or put some food up high. However, it is not always seen as the strongest knot and it is not something that you are able to use for heavy jobs, such as stringing a hammock between the trees.
- Figure eight: The basic figure eight knot is the stopper knot. This means that it is going to be tied at the end of a rope to keep it from sliding through a hole. It is sometimes used as a basic knot because it is a bit stronger compared to the bowline and will be able to hold onto more weight.
- Double figure eight: This is the knot that you will use to link two ropes together, even if they are not the same size. You will first

make the basic figure eight knot and then you would follow the path of the original figure eight knot with the new rope.

It is a good idea to learn how to work with these different knots so that you are able to prepare in case something comes up.

Natural shelters

There will be some times when you will not be able to find the right materials or you do not have enough time to make the shelter before it gets dark. When this happens, you will want to go for on that is naturally occurring. This is going to vary based on where you get lost. For example, if you get lost in a wooded area, you may want to look for a hollow log to work with. This will allow you to get inside and then cover the entrance with leaves and other materials to make sure that the cold is kept out. Make sure to look for wasp or bee nests inside before getting started. If that is not possible, you can work with some pine needles to cover yourself or a depression in the ground to make a shelter.

There are some places in the country that will have rock or caves that will work to protect you from the rain or snow. However, it is important to make sure tat you are not sharing your space with another animal. This could lead to a really bad encounter, no matter where you are in the world.

If you need to use a cave or a rock overhanging for your shelter, then you must not build a fire. Sometimes the rocks that are inside of these areas can break off if you heat them too much. This does not mean that you have to go without a fire if you choose these as your natural shelter. Just make sure that you build the fire outside of the overhand and the cover, rather than inside.

If you are in the part of the country where there are some mines, it is important to stay away from them. there are gases in mines that can kill you off if you breathe in the air. There are also a lot of animals that are inside these mines such as scorpions, rattlesnakes, and mountain lions. And these mines are going to be unstable and the floors could fall out from under you or the ceilings may fall on you. They may look like a good idea, but they are so dangerous so pick out a different shelter.

Tarp shelters

Another idea that you can go with is a tarp shelter. This is a good choice if you are in an area that is warm and you would like to protect yourself from the rain or build up some shade in the heat. If you did not bring a tarp along with you, it is fin to work with one of the trash bags that you bring along. You can just cut it open on the long side and then make it into on large plastic sheet. There are a lot of ways that you are able to build this kind of shelter and the way that you do this will depend on what is available all around you.

The first option is to use a clove hitch knot so that you can tie the top corners of the tarp between two bushes or two trees and then stretch out the tarp between them. You can then pull the bottom edge of your tarp out and down to make a half tent and set down something heavy, like logs, rocks, or sand to keep the corners in place.

It is also possible to fold the tarp into a diagonal and then tie one corner of the fold to an overhanging branch with the help of the bowline knot and then hold down on your edges with some rocks. This will create an open-end tent. If you have your survival kit on you and your tube tent is inside, it is going to be good to create a tarp shelter quickly. This tube tent is going to be open-ended plastic tent will already have a rope and it is easy to carry around with you.

Trench shelters

You can also consider working with trench shelters. This is a basic shelter that is good for helping you to deal with cold and warm weather. You will be able to build this kind of shelter in the sand or snow and since they can be done with your hands, it does not matter how many tools you have on you. the steps that you should follow to make one of these trench shelters includes:

- Dig out a pit, soft dirt, sand or piling snow around the edges so that it is deeper. You only want to make it big enough that you are able to lie down. Leave a small opening to make it easier to slide down into the shelter.
- Make the bed you will sleep on at the bottom of the pit. Line this with lots of bark, leaves, and pine branches so you are not on top of wet ground.
- On top of the shelter, add some sticks and branches to make a roof. Add a garbage bag or tarp on this if you have one.
- Cover the top of the roof you just made with some branches, pine needles, leaves, snow, or anything else that is nearby so that you can seal it up.

- When this is done, slide into the trench, using your feet first, and then close the entrance. Leave just enough opening so you get fresh air, but close up the rest to keep you warm.

Brush shelters

Sometimes you may need to create a brush shelter. This is a good one to learn about because it is easy to construct and can be made in most environments. You will not need to dig into the ground and it is a good one if you need to conserve energy. The steps you can follow to make a brush shelter include the following:

- Find a dead tree that is still pretty sturdy and let this be the central support of the shelter. It should be about three or four feet bigger than you, but still small enough that you are able to list and move it. Break off the sharp branches that are sticking out of it.
- Pick a secure place to prop up the pole. It should be a place that is four feet off the ground and somewhat lat. The spot can be a place on a tree where the two branches come together, for example. Lay the narrower part of the ridgepole against this flat spot and the

wider end can go on the ground. If you have some cord on you, tie the ridgepole to the surface you chose to make it more secure.
- Gather your materials to use as bedding and carry them back to the shelter. Consider carrying them in a trash bag to make things easier.
- Make your bed under the ridgepole, stretch it out, and then check to see if you fit in there. You may need to adjust things a bit.
- Drape your tarp over the ridgepole to make a type of tent and secure all the sides down with some rocks.
- Fill in the frame with some more branches, bark, and sticks. You can weave together smaller branches to help it all hold together. You want to use all the material you can to cover all the shelter except the entrance.
- When everything is covered up, it is time to work on the shelter door. You can use a bag full of leaves, pile up branches, or use your backpack to help keep things out of the shelter.

These are just some of the shelters that you are able to work with when it comes to surviving when you get lost. It will often depend on your location when you get lost and what materials are close to you at the time. if you are able to, consider trying out a few of these shelter types so you are prepared when it is time to survive in the wilderness.

Chapter 6: How to Stay Safe From Wild Animals

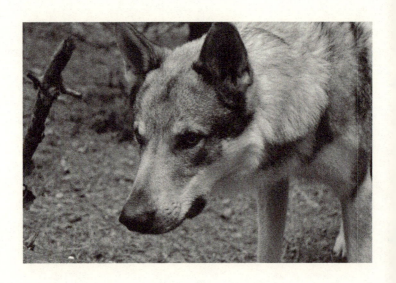

When you are on the trail, it is important to note that there are a lot of animals out there. These are wild animals who have made the wilderness their friend, and you need to figure out the best way to stay safe. For many kids, the scariest thing about being lost out in the middle of nowhere at night is the thought of a dangerous animal, predator, or even snakes that may get them. You may wonder if it is safe to stay in your shelter, what you should do if you see a dangerous animal, or how safe you really are.

The first thing to realize is that you should just relax. Although there are some times when a wild animal will attack a human, these are really are. Many people are scared about mountain lions (it doesn't help that there are thousands of these animals in the meadows, woods, and some neighborhoods), but there have only been about 20 people in over 100 years who have ben killed by one in the United States.

When you hear those scary noises outside your shelter at night, it is not likely that those noises are from dangerous animals. The rustling sound you hear is most likely from a mouse, raccoon, or deer.

In the case where there is something more dangerous out the door, you should take some deep breaths and remain calm. Thousands of people see and hear dangerous animals each year, but none of them get attacked so you are safe.

If you are someone who likes to go out and hike on a regular basis, it is likely that you pass by dangerous animals on a regular basis and you do not even know it. The reason that you don't see these dangerous animals and you are not harmed in the process is because you are not engaging in activities that will put you in danger. You also know that when you do come across a wild animal, it is a good idea to be prepared for an emergency.

It is a good idea to know what animals are out there in any area you plan to travel. You can learn all the wildlife, including which animals may be dangerous, what you are able to do if you come across one, and the best ways to just stay away from those animals. To start, let's take a look at some of the simple rules you should follow when you encounter any wild animal when you are lost:

- Leave the animal alone: You must always give the wild animal some space. Most animals you encounter, even the ones who are dangerous, simply want to get away from you. move out of the way. Do not try to get closer or take a picture or do something else to provoke the animal, or you risk getting bitten or worse. It does not matter if the animal is one you considered dangerous or it looks harmless, just leave the animals along.

- Bring some protection: If you hike in areas that have lots of bears, consider bringing some bear spray. This will have some hot peppers in it and is designed to keep some of those larger dangerous animals away. A large walking stick can be used to scare away mountain lions, bears, and coyotes. You can also use these to check the tall grasses around you for snakes. A small air horn is not only good for signaling to others where you are, but they will keep the mountain lions and bears away.

- Use your instincts: While you are out, keep in tune with your feelings. If you have a dog with you, pay attention to their behavior as well. These could be signs that a dangerous animal is nearby.

- Look around: It is not a good idea to just look in one direction when you hike. Check all around you to see if there are wild animals. This includes forwards, behind you, up ledges and rock piles, and even in trees. Learn some animal tracks and look out for some signs of a predator that look new. These will help you to determine if there is a dangerous animal near you.

It is important that you always look around you and notice what is going on with your surroundings. This will ensure that you are careful about the dangerous animals, that you are aware when they are near you, and that you are giving them the space that they need.

Mountain lions

Mountain lions go by a variety of names including catamount, panther, wildcat, cougar, and puma. These are large cats that can weight hundreds of pounds and have the ability to jump up to 20 feet. They have a diet of deer for the most part. Inside the United States, these animals live in the Southwest, Great Plains, and the West Coast, although you can find them in Mexico and in parts of Canada. But even when you live in these areas, it is likely that you will never even see a mountain lion. Their numbers are large, but they usually like to hide away from people.

Mountain lions like to follow anything that is moving quickly, such as animals, bike riders, and runners. They will really go after something that breaks out into a run suddenly, which is something you may be tempted to do when you see a lion, to little kids moving around, and to dogs.

If you are hiking in a mountain lion area, it is important to look behind you frequently while you are walking. Look at the hills, trees, and ledges as well. If you find a fresh kill, especially if it is a dead deer, it is time to get out of the area since mountain lions usually stay near their kill. Keep the dog close to you and make sure that you are in a group.

When you encounter a mountain lion, never turn your back on it, never bend over or crouch down, and do not try to run away from the lion. You should not run, scream or panic either. These things will just make the situation a lot worse.

The way that you react will depend on the actions of the mountain lion. If the lion is far away and doesn't seem to be paying much attention to you, your danger level is low. Make sure that you stay in a group, that your eyes are on the lion, and you do not block the lions exit. You also do not want to start talking excitedly or run around and catch the attention of the lion.

If the lion is following you and watching you, but it is more than fifty yards from you, the danger is medium for adults but higher for kids. This means that the lion is curios about you. you should not try to kneel down, bend over or turn your back. Find a rock or a stick that you can grab without bending down. Stand up straight and make yourself look as big as you can. If you are in an area where you can do it, it is time to back away as slowly as possible.

Now, if the lion is staring at you and they are less than fifty yards away, then the risk is high. At this point, the lion is wondering if it is going to attack you. If you have the ability to get into a car, then this is something you should do.

If you are near a mountain lion and it is crouching or crawling to you with its tail twitching and it has its eyes on you intently, then your risk level is really high. At this point, the lion is looking for a way to attack you. if you have a rock, it is time to throw it or to bring out that pepper spray. You can also make scary faces, show your teeth, or growl. You should never get your eyes off the lion and you should never move to lower ground.

Finally, if the lions ears are flattened down and it has its rear legs moving up or down or doing a pumping motion, the lion is abut to attack. It is time to defend yourself. There are some times when you can stop the attack by rushing at the lion with a stick that is raised up like a weapon. If the lion is right by you, poke it in the mouth and the eyes with your stick, but make sure that you are not near the teeth and paws.

Bears

For the most part, people have become smarter about bears. They know that they should not leave any food around their shelters that may attract the bears. Hikers know that they should leave their food high up to keep them away from the food and you should not wear lotions that smell like food.

The biggest reason that bears are going to attack people is because they are startled when they meet up with that person. When you are out in bear country, make some noise to warn the bear so they know you are there. Bear bells will help or you can clap your hands and yell every few minutes. Be careful when you are near a noisy area, like a creek, because it is harder for a bear to hear you.

Some bears will attack because they feel hungry or the mother bear is worried that her cubs will be in danger. This means that if you want to stay safe in bear country, you must make sure that you avoid bears or you reassure them that you will not pose a threat to them or the cubs.

Any time that you see a bear, it is time to leave the area because there is not much warning when a bear wants to attack. If you see that the bear is swaying their heads, clacking their teeth, or huffing noises, it is time to get out of the way. When the bear stands on its hind legs, they are trying to see you better.

Most bears will be attracted to the smell of food. If you are lost in bear country, it is a good idea to cook at a place that is about 50 yards from your shelter if that is possible. No food item should be near your camp so that you don't attract a bear over there. You also should keep the smell of food off your clothes and avoid wearing any fruity-smelling soap, perfume, shampoo, sunscreen, or lip balm.

To make sure that your food and yourself are safe, make sure that you hang the food from a tree and have it about 50 yards from the shelter. The food should be placed in a sturdy bag or wrap it up before tying it to the tree. The food should be hung at least 12 feet of the ground and 10 feet from the tree to keep it safe.

Again, the way that you react to a bear is going to depend on the actions that you see with the bear. If the bear is still some distance away from you and not paying that much attention you should turn around and backtrack along the trail. You should walk about 15 minutes and then take another trail. If you need to go back to that same trail where you saw the bear the bear, wait another 20 minutes before you go.

If you see that the bear is nearby or on the trail with you, but it is not close enough to really notice you, then you should back away from the bear, while keeping your eyes on them. you can get out the bear spray if it is on you, and then keep moving backwards. You should not make eye contact, but back away 400 yards.

If the bear gets to close range, it is important to not scream, run, or panic. These actions will cause the bear to attack. It is better to talk soothingly to the bear, but do not bend over or make eye contact with the bear. Back away if you notice that the bear is not acting aggressively. If you see that the activity you are doing upsets the bear, it is time to stop moving.

Now if the bear starts to charge you, it is still important that you do not panic. Most charges from a bear will be a bluff. If the bear doesn't stop, spray them with a pepper spray. If you don't have your spray, drop some item, such as your hat, and then back away. This can be a distraction to the bear and they may be willing to stop and examine it. Do not use your food or pack for this because you will not get it back.

And finally, if a bear starts to attack you, it is important to know how to handle it. Most bears will only attack as a defensive move. Once a bear decides that you are not a threat, it will leave. It is better to curl up into a ball, making sure to cover your head and neck with your arms and play dead. If your pack is on, lie down on your stomach with the pack on your back for protection. Do not move until you are sure the bear is gone.

Take care of going to the bathroom when it comes to wildlife

If you explore the outdoors, it is a good idea to bring hand sanitizer and toilet paper with you. When picking out an area to use as a bathroom, you should pick an area that is far away from your shelter. Human urine and feces can draw in the mountain lions and bears to your camp. Smaller animals will come as well because they are attracted to the minerals that are in it.

When you are in the woods, it is best to dig a hole and then cover it up when you are done going to the bathroom. If you are able to use a river or a lake instead, this is even better. Moving water will ensure that the scent will go away from you. Even if you are not able to find a river to do this, make sure that your bathroom is about 100 yards away from the camp. Go with a direction where the wind will not blow any scent toward the camp. This helps to keep your area clean, but it can help to keep the predator animals away from your camp.

Wolves

Another wild animal that you should deal with is wolves. These animals are generally going to be shy and they are happy to avoid humans. If you are in wolf country, it is a good idea to let the wolves know that you are in the area by clapping and making noise. Wolves are much more likely to attack a dog rather than you. It is also not likely that you will see a wild wolf, but if one does come around, it is a good idea to make yourself tall and big, throw things at them, yell, and back away. You should not make eye contact with the wolf. If it continues to approach you, keep looking big, throwing things, and yell to show that you are too dangerous for the wolf to attack you.

Coyotes

Just like with wolves, coyotes are going to be afraid of people. It is likely that you will be able to scare them away by yelling, throwing sticks, and making lots of loud noises. Since the 1800s, there have only been about 30 coyote attacks on humans in the United States, and most of these victims were not hurt that bad. If you are in an area that has a lot of coyotes, it is important that you do not leave food outside because this is a big reason why coyotes will attack.

Although these attacks by coyotes on humans are pretty rare, they are more likely to go for children rather than adults. Coyotes also like cats and dogs for good. sometimes the coyote will try to get the dog away from you before the whole pack goes after them.

Venomous snakes

Each year, there are hundreds of snakes that are actually harmless that are killed because people are not able to tell the difference between a venomous snake and a nonvenomous one. Inside the United

States, there are only four dangerous species of snakes that you will need to watch out for. These snakes include the following:

- Rattlesnakes: In most states, these are the only snake you will need to worry about. You are able to find rattlesnakes almost anywhere. All rattlesnakes are going to have a thick body and triangular head, but of course, the best way to recognize the rattle on their tails.
- Copperheads: These are colorful snakes are found in the eastern and southern states, in forest and swampy areas. They are sometimes invisible when they coil among the leaves and they will freeze up when people are near them. they come with triangular heads and thick bodies like the rattlesnake, but their color pattern will be different.
- Cottonmouths or water moccasins: There is only one venomous water snake in the United States, and that is the water moccasin. These are harder to identify because they can come in various patterns and colors. Some people see these as aggressive, but it is your job to move away and avoid them as much as possible.

- Coral snakes: These are related to cobras and are found in the southern part of the United States. These snakes must chew on their victims to inject the venom so the bites are not as dangerous as the others.

All of the snakes you may encounter will want to be left alone. Most of the life-threatening snake bites could be prevented if you made sure to leave a snake alone. Always watch your hands and feet, especially when you are walking around on a warm evening (this is when they like to hunt) or when you are moving around rocks.

If a snake does end up biting you, stay calm. The first thing to do is see if it was a venomous variety. If the bite is from a nonvenomous sake, clean out the wound and bandage it. Even if you are bitten by a venomous snake, it is unlikely that you will dy. This is because one out of four snake bites made by a venomous snake is a dry bite, which means that the snake failed to inject that dangerous venom at all. However, if you do get some venom in you, some of the symptoms you should watch for include:

- Increased saliva
- Sweating
- Trouble breathing

- Dizziness or nausea
- Severe pain
- Swelling and lots of redness in the bite area
- Changes in vision,
- Numbness
- Fever
- Thirst
- Tingling in your body or face

It is best to get help as soon as possible if this happens. Stay calm and get away from the snake. If you get upset and start to get nervous, this can make the venom move around much faster and could make the situation worse. Some things that you should consider doing instead include:

- Take off any jewelry that you have near the site right away.
- Take off your tight-fitting clothes that are near the site of the bite
- Do not add ice to the bite area
- Do not take any medication that is meant to relieve pain.
- Do not cut across the fang marks and try to suck out the poison.
- Do not use a tourniquet to stop the blood flow to where the bite is.
- Get to the hospital as soon as you can.

The best thing to do against snake bites is to prevent them from happening. It helps to stay aware of where you place your hands and feet and always watch your surroundings so that these bites will not happen in the first place.

Chapter 7: First Aid Tips to Keep You Safe

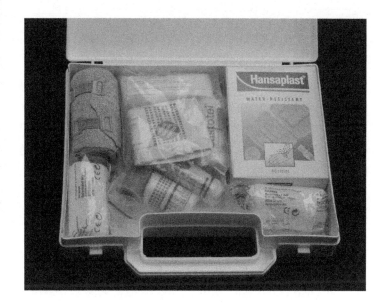

It is important that you know how to take care of yourself if you get lost. Things can happen, such as falling on the trail or touching some poison ivy and you will need to take care of things until someone can get there to help you out. This chapter is going to take some time to look at the first aid tools and tips that you can use to make sure that you are safe at all times.

Building your first aid kit

If you plan to go out into the wilderness to hike, it is a good idea to bring your own first aid kit with you. This should be lightweight and easy to fit into your bag, but make sure that it has all the items that my may need in case you get harmed or injured. Some of the things that you should consider adding into your first aid kit include:

- Disposable gloves: If you need to handle bodily fluids, burns, or wounds, wear some gloves. This will keep you from getting diseases or infecting the area.

- Gauze pads or some kind of tissue: These are good to clean out a wound before you use any antiseptic on it.
- Antiseptic wipes: These are the best to use because they will not take up all that much space in your bag, but can help to clean some cuts and scrapes that you have. These will come in little packets and you should use them to clean out a wound before you bandage it up. Some are pain-free, but most will contain some alcohol and will sting a bit.
- Antibiotic ointment: You will put this on a cut or wound to ensure that it does not become infected. These are not going to sting, but will keep you safe. You can purchase these in tiny packets or in a tube.
- Adhesive bandages: These are also known as Band-Aids. They will keep your smaller wounds covered and cleaned. Pick out some different sizes and shapes to meet all your needs.
- Butterfly bandages: These are small but strong adhesive bandages that are in the shape of a butterfly. They are good for holding deeper cuts closed and to stop bleeding. Pinch the cut closed and then tape it tightly across the wound.
- Elastic bandage (rolled): These are also known as Ace bandage. You would use them

to wrap up an injured joint, like your wrist or the ankles.
- Medical adhesive tape: There are some different options to choose from here, but you should get the type that is easy to tear by hand to avoid carrying scissors.
- Hand sanitizer
- Hydrocortisone cream: This can be used to help out with any kind of skin reaction. You can use them with poison ivy, stings, but bites, swelling, redness, and itchiness.
- Antihistamine or your EpiPen: Many people will carry Benadryl because it helps to stop some allergic reactions that you will get from stings or bites. This will make you a bit sleepy, but it can be a lifesaver. If you or someone else who is on the trail with you is really allergic to bee stings or something else, you should consider having an EpiPen on you in case.
- Stomach soothing pills
- Pain relief tablets: These can be nice if you are injured, burnt, or break a bone. It is best to avoid aspirin though. Go with Advil, Motrin, Aleve, or Tylenol.
- Sling: You can buy a sling with safety pins to attach it together. This will be helpful if you have an arm injury or you can use it as an ankle brace.

- Tweezers: Splinters are something that you will often need to deal with. Tweezers will help to remove the splinter, as well as removing ticks if needed.
- Needle: This can help you to sew parts of your shelter together, or for getting splinters out from underneath the skin.
- Aloe vera lotion: This is a great thing to have along if you are going to be out in the hot sun all day. It is a plant based lotion that is known to sooth your skin if it has been irritated or if it got sunburnt.

If there is anything else that you think you will need to help with a particular medical problem or something else, make sure that you add it to your first aid kit. These first aid kits can be customized so you are able to put in exactly what you need to stay safe.

Doing some basic first aid when lost

Hopefully, you will be able to stay safe when you are on the trail and can wait it out until someone is able to find you. While this is usually what happens, you never know when something small, such as spraining your ankle or something else, can make you go down while you are lost.

It is so important that you have at least the basics when it comes to first aid in the wild and that you know how you are supposed to apply them, even if the situation is stressful. Even knowing how you are able to treat some pretty minor injuries will help to make a difference in an emergency situation. It at least helps you to treat minor injuries and will make it easier for you to keep some of the more serious casualties stable until someone can get to you to help.

Now, there are a ton of ailments and injuries that could potentially affect you. We will not have time to go through all of them, but as long as you know some of the basic principles that come with first aid, you will be able to use those to help you out no matter what the situation may be.

First, there will be some first aid priorities that you must assess. You will need to start by checking if there is any danger around you or if you are going to be in more danger if you stop right there to fix the issue. You should not move yourself or the other person if you are not sure of the injuries, unless there is more danger in staying put than moving. If necessary, try to make the area as safe as possible, but do not cause any more harm than necessary. If you are helping someone else, do not move them if they have a spinal or neck injuries, unless you must because they are having difficulties with breathing.

Then you need to check the breathing of the person. Check that their airway is open and that they are breathing. A person who is unconscious is not going to have control over their muscles so you must be careful to keep the tongue from obstructing the airways. The airway is usually cleared out with a simple method of tilting the chin and head up gently. This helps to pull the tongue away from the air passages.

Once they are breathing, you can place the unconscious and breathing person in a recovery position. You can move them to the side, with the uppermost leg at a right angle from the body. Support the head by the hand of the uppermost arm. You should check to makes sure that the head is tilted back a bit so that the airways will remain clear. Of course, if you think that the other person has a spine or neck injury, then don't do anything at all.

Now you will take a look at the bleeding that is going on. You should stop any bleeding. All external bleeding, even open wounds, will be treated using the same method. The steps that you should do for this include the following:

- Squeeze together the sides of the wound. Use your finger to apply direct pressure on the wound, but working with sterile dressing is better. Some clean clothing will work if you do not have any other options.
- Lie the casualty down
- Lift the wounded part so that it is above the level of the heart. This works because it slows down the breathing.
- Bandage the wound. You want to make sure it is done firmly, but do not cut off the circulation to that area.

If you look at the other person and you feel that the injury is going to cause internal bleeding, the first thing that you should do is figure out how to prevent the shock from occurring. It is important to get medical attention for this as soon as possible.

And finally, you should watch out for shock in the other person. Shock is going to be a condition of general weakness in the body, and it is going to be present in all kinds of accidents, although it will show up in different degrees and ways. When shock hits, you or the other person may feel giddy, restless, anxious, faint, or weak. Keep the other person quiet and warm and try to be as reassuring as you can.

The most important thing that you can do to keep yourself safe is to bring along your first aid kit. This will help you out so much more than trying to make due when you are out in the middle of nowhere and it can really make sure that you are going to keep small issues from taking over.

Chapter 8: How to Deal with Bugs on the Trail

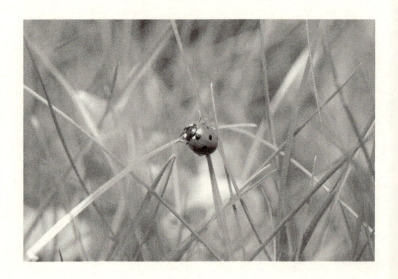

Although your biggest concerns may be those mountain lions and bears, the bugs around you can often prove more dangerous to your health when you are out on the trail. This is mainly because those tiny bugs are carrying some big diseases. However this is not an excuse to be scared of all the bugs you encounter. This chapter will look at some of the bugs you need to watch out for and will show you the steps to take to avoid them and stay safe.

Mosquitoes

Anyone who has made it through a summer knows how annoying mosquitoes are. They like to follow you around and bite so you are itching all day long. But not only do these insects bite you and leave a ton of itchy spots all over, these bugs will carry diseases on them as well. Just in the United States, mosquitoes can be infected with West Nile virus and several types of encephalitis.

The good news is that mosquito carried illnesses in the United States are pretty rare. And most of us have been bitten by these bugs without having more than some mild irritation at the bite spot. With some good insect repellent, you can move your risk so that it is practically not there.

When you plan to be outside, especially when it is hot out or you will be near some standing water make sure that you use insect repellent and that you use it any time that a mosquito is around. If you happen to be lost and you do not have this repellent, it is a good idea to cover your body with a tarp or extra clothing and then add on a layer of mud to any areas of the body that are exposed. If you planned to go out ahead of time, consider taking a bit of mosquito netting to put over your head to protect from any swarm of mosquitoes that may come around.

When a bug bites you, it can become swollen, hurt, and really itch. Scratching at the itch is just going to make the situation worse. It is better to pull out some hydrocortisone cream so that you can lessen the swelling, redness, and itching that you get from these bug bites.

Ticks

No one likes to deal with ticks. These ticks will be found in rural areas throughout the United States, except at the very highest altitudes. Some ticks are really small and will only be the size of a sesame seed. They will have tiny heads, large bodies, and eight legs. They are able to attach themselves to animals and humans and will suck their blood. Then they work to drop off and lay eggs to help make more ticks. These little bugs are able to infect you with up to 11 different diseases which include Lyme disease, anaplasmosis, relapsing fever, and Rocky Mountain spotted fever.

The best way that you are able to keep these ticks off you are to spray your clothing with insect repellent. Wearing a hat, long sleeves, and long pants can help. Consider tucking your pant legs into your hiking boots. This will help to make it harder for the ticks to gain access to your skin.

Ticks are going to be fund in wooded and grassy areas with lots of busses and sometimes they will be found in places where deer have made beds in the grass and leaves. They will be more active when it s summer, but it is possible to run across them no matter what time of year.

To avoid these ticks when you are lost, stay at the middle of the trail and try as much as you can to avoid brushing against grasses or bushes. It is common to pick up ticks by sitting on a stump or a log, so check the area before you sit down. After you are ready to set up camp for the night, inspect yourself to see if any ticks hitched a ride. Look around the ears, in your hair, behind the knees, around your waist, and even under the arms. These ticks can hide anywhere that is easy to miss when you glance around.

Despite the common advice that you may be given, you should not use Vaseline or a lit match to get rid of a tick. This is just going to get the tick to inject some more saliva into you, causing you to get much sicker. Instead, you should remove it by the hand, while wearing gloves or some tissue, or work with some tweezers. Grab the tick close to your skin and then pull it up and away from the skin. Never twist it. When the tick is out, clean up that area with some antiseptic.

If you found a tick on you and you then feel sick for days or weeks after the bite of the tick, it is time to visit your doctor to get seen. There are some treatments that you are able to use when it comes to tick diseases, but these are going to work the best the sooner you take them after you feel sick.

Chiggers

Chiggers are little red mites that have the ability to bite you and then cause some terrible itching. They are not going to burrow down into your skin.

Instead, they will be able to crawl up your clothing before they start to bite you. To keep chiggers off you, it is best to tuck your pants into your boots or your socks or use some insect repellent. You will usually find these chiggers in damp and hot areas, but it is less likely that you will see these insects if you are in the desert or in the mountains.

Ants

Most of the ants that you will encounter are harmless. But there are some, such as red harvester ants and fire ants, that can be bad. These insects are known to attack and will repeatedly sting pets, birds, animals, and people. When you are stung, the ant will be able to inject a poison that will make the skin feel like it is on fire. That poison is even able to cause some blisters to show up on the skin, and some people are even allergic so one bite could not only hurt, but it could cause issues with breathing and some other medical issues.

Although the fire ant is not a native animal in the United States, they have spread through the country rapidly. These bugs prefer to be in the suburban areas, especially those with cleared grounds, but it is possible to find them in logs and under rocks as well. Fire ants are known for climbing into your clothes and then stinging you over and over again.

If you are stung by a fire ant, you need to wash of that area to help remove the poison that is on the skin. You should use some cold water to help keep the swelling down and then use some hydrocortisone cream to reduce the swelling.

When it comes to the read harvester ants, you can be bitten and stung. These ants are a reddish color as well and they will live in holes that are left behind by plats and grass. Cow killers are another type of ant that you must look out for. This ant is more of a red, yellow, or orange and many say that the sting is so painful on these, that it is one of the worst that you can get from any insect in North America.

For being so small, these insects can pack on a powerful sting that hurts. The key to avoiding the ant attacks is to leave the ants lone. Before you start on your shelter, check to see if there are any ants that are there. If you do see some of these ants, it is better to move away and find somewhere else to build your shelter.

Wasps and bees

Coming across a bee can be a scary experience. Most of the bees you will encounter are honeybees and these are not going to sting you unless you step on them, swat at them, or do something else that will upset them. Killer bees are a bit different because they are able to attack pets and people without a good reason or warning.

You will not be able to tell the difference between a killer bee ad a good bee just from looking at them. This means that if you see a beehive, it is best to avoid it and move out of the area to stay safe.

If you are out on the trail and you are being attacked by a swarm of bees, the best thing to do is run. Bees are only willing to follow you so far, so keep on running until you can get them to stop chasing you, or you reach some kind of shelter that will keep you safe. It is not wise to jump into water because bees may wait around and will attack as soon as you come up for water. Bees are known to be attracted to movement so do not swat at them. Trying to kill them is even worse. If you kill one, they will release a scent that will attract other angry bees and the situation just gets worse.

Some bees will have a barbed stinger that will break off as soon as they sting you. When you are safe, you can remove the stinger as long as you do not squeeze on it because this will release more venom. You can use something flat, like a knife or a key, to help get the stingers out. cold cloths and ice packs are good for reducing the pain and swelling. If none of those are available, hold the area that was stung underwater to help or cover with some cool mud. If you have it on you, some hydrocortisone cream may help. For those who are allergic to bee stings make sure that you have your EpiPen on you at all times when you are hiking.

While you are last, you may have to deal with wasps. These do not produce honey or rely on pollen and flower nectar. These insects will nest in trees, on the ground and old buildings and they are not scared to attack if you get too close to their nest. They will not lose their stingers, so they are able to sting you as many times as they want. The most aggressive wasp type that you should watch out for is the yellow jacket. These yellow jackets are attracted to food from humans so keep this cleaned up as much as you can.

Kissing bugs

Kissing bugs are found in the warmer areas of the United States. These winged insects will look like beetles and will bite you at night before sucking your blood. They are black or brown in color and will be small; no more than an inch long. You will be able to find them near rodents' nests. They belong to a group of insects that is known as assassin bugs. Their bites will cause a wide variety of reactions that range from itchy welts on the body or face to a swollen tongue and trouble breathing.

There are some people who will have life-threatening reactions to these bites. Even if you are not allergic to them, if you are bitten by a few of these, you may experience some more severe reactions at the later bites.

Scorpions

You must also watch out for scorpions. These are found on any terrain and they come with eight legs, two pincers on the front, and a thick and long tail that has a stinger on the end. There are many kinds, but the only one that is considered dangerous is the Arizona bark scorpion. All types of scorpions will sting you if you provoke them. they live under rocks and inside of logs that are rotted, so you should take care when you are looking for your firewood. They will usually come out of their homes only at night and can crawl into your shoes while you are sleeping. Make sure to check your clothes, and especially your shoes, when you wake up.

A sting from a scorpion should be treated in the same manner as a bee sting. You will scrape of the stinger if one was left behind and then add some cold water or ice to that area. If you are stung by a scorpion and you start to have trouble breathing, have extreme pain, or you have a sensation that eels like electrical jolts at the site of the sting, it is time to find help immediately.

Spiders

While there are more than 2000 people who report a venomous spider bite each year in the United States, only four are killed by one of these spider bites each year. While there are many spiders who have bites that are painful there are only four that will be considered dangerous. These include:

- Black widows: These spiders will hide under logs, bushes, and rocks and in cool and dark places. Many bites have occurred in outhouses for example. They may also hide in your shoes at night as well. If you get a bite from a black widow, there is a change that you will not develop symptoms at all. There are cases where the venom will be able to create painful and severe muscle cramps.

- Brown widows: These are the relatives of the black widow and they are not native n the United States. Some say that these are not as dangerous as a black widow, but they are still ones that you need to be careful for.
- Brown recluse spiders: These are small spiders that are found in the Midwestern United States. They are sometimes called violin spiders because of the markings that are found at the top of their bodies. They often match the other varieties of brown spiders so it is best to just leave them all alone.
- Hobo spiders: Hobo spider bites are going to sometimes be confused with brown recluse spiders since the bites are similar between the two. They are small to medium size and will spin some webs that are funnel-shaped.

A bite from any of the above could harm you. In fact, if you end up getting bit at all, it is best to seek medical help because it is hard to tell from a glance whether the spider is dangerous or not. You will usually know quickly if you were bitten because you will feel pain or some itching right after. With some of the spiders, such as with the black widow or a brown widow, you will feel a bit sick, and get a fever and headache or a terrible back or stomach pain. When this happens, you need to go see your doctor and get some antivenom to help you. Place some cold water on the bite to help you out until you are able to get yourself over to a hospital.

There are some spiders that will seem more threatening than they really are and you will not need to worry about them as much. Tarantulas are a good example of this and they are large, hairy, and will look scary, but they are not venomous. Although they will bite if you provoke them, they are usually going to be docile to you.

There are a lot of insects you will need to be careful about when you are out in the wild. For being so small, they can cause a lot of issues, such as pain and getting sick it is important to be aware of what is going on around you and leave these insects alone. Doing this will make it easier for you to stay safe.

Chapter 9: Tips About Foraging for Food

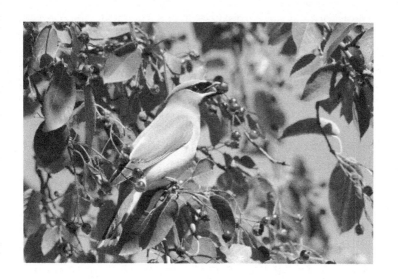

To be honest, if you are lost in the wilderness, you may not spend that much time looking for food. Your first priorities will be to get some water and build up a shelter. Then you will move on to signaling for others to come find you so you can go home. You may even have some food on you already and will be able to make it the few days before someone finds you without needing to look around for food at all.

It is still a good idea to know how to forage for your own food. There may be a reason that people will not be able to get to you as quickly as they would like, and being able to find your own food will make all the difference. It is a good thing to know how to forage for edible plants, and how to trap and kill wild game. Sure, it is smart to bring along some food with you, such as dehydrated meals, trail mix, and jerky, but if you get lost without having these supplies, it is much better to be prepared.

Before we get into this, one piece of advice that you should follow is to ignore the old saying that you are able to eat anything if you see that an animal is eating it. This is not true. There are bugs that are able to eat mushrooms that are deadly to humans. Goats can eat poison oak, along with some other plants, that would make you extremely ill. Garter snakes can eat some salamanders that are poisonous and would kill a human adult in just a few hours.

Plants to avoid

To start with, it is important to know which plants you should not eat at all. In addition to plenty of edible plants, the wilderness is filled with many plants that may make you sick or may kill you in a few hours after you eat them. Most poisonous plants will have similar characteristics. It is important to not eat or touch any plant that has the following:

- Sap that is milky or changes color when you cut open the plant, such as going from clear to white.
- Clusters of flowers that make an umbrella
- Bulbs that look similar to an onion or garlic
- Carrot-like roots and leaves
- Seeds that are pink, black or purple
- Plants that smell like almonds
- Single berries, especially if they are red, yellow, green or white ones
- Leaves that have tiny hairs or fuzz on them.
- Bean-like pods or plants that have parts that look like peas

There are several different plants that you must avoid if you would like to keep from getting sick when you are lost. Some of the most common types include the following:

Mushrooms

Each year, there are about 8000 people who become poisoned by eating mushrooms. The majority of these people do not die, but they can do some damage to their liver or kidneys. Most edible mushrooms will look almost the same to their poisonous relatives, so this may be a good type that you avoid. It is best to avoid mushrooms, as well as their fungi, because while some are safe, it is too hard to tell the difference between them.

Death camas

These are sometimes known as black snakeroot and it is found in natural areas and meadows in the United States. These little bulbs will look like wild onions, and they often grow right next to them so it is hard to tell the difference. The best way to know is that onions are going to smell like onions, but death camas will not. They also have leaves that are a little bit different, but they are still hard to tell apart. This death camas is one of the most poisonous plants in nature and it has been responsible for the death of livestock across the country. Eating just one flower or bulb could kill you in a few hours. When you are in the wilderness, it is best to avoid any onion looking plant to be safe.

Hemlock

Hemlock is one of those plants that you should not touch or eat. It is a flowering plant that has flowers that grow together in umbrella clusters. It is found in meadows and in damp areas. The root looks like a wild carrot or parsnip and sometimes it is hard to tell the difference between them and hemlock. Since there are quite a few plants that look like hemlock, it is best to avoid any plants that are similar.

Bean or pea type plants

Many plants that are really toxic are going to have seedpods that look like a bean or some wild peas. If you are out on the trail and notice that there is something that has a bean or a pea that is growing on it, it is best to leave it alone.

Nettles

Nettles and other plants that contain hairy or fuzzy leaves, can sometimes cause stinging burns if you touch them and some will have toxins that will make you sick if you decide to eat them. It is possible to eat nettles as long as you properly boil them in water, but it is usually best to leave them alone. If you are stung by one of these plants, it is possible to treat that sting like you would with a bee sting.

Berries

When it comes to berries, you must be careful. Unless you know for sure that these berries are safe, it is best to just leave them alone. Some common plants that will also have poisonous berries include yews, jimson weed, deadly nightshade, mistletoe, and holly. Most single berries will be dangerous to eat, so unless you know exactly what you are looking for, it is best to leave these alone. Always avoid green, yellow, or white single berries. However, if you see aggregate berries, or ones where the fruit is made up of lots of tiny berries, these are edible and you can enjoy. Some examples of these would be thimbleberries, raspberries, and blackberries.

Poison oak, ivy, and sumac

Although these are all going to look different, all three of these plants will be the same in that they contain poisonous oils that will cause a rash when your skin touches them. You may be exposed to these by directly touching the plant, but it can also cause a problem if you touch something that brushed up against the plant, such as if your jacket or an animal rubbed up against you. Each of these plants can have a different appearance, which makes them hard to identify.

If you do end up touching one of these plants, it is a good idea to keep some hydrocortisone cream in your bag. This can be so great at helping to soothe the itch that you have and at calming down the reaction that your skin has to the poisonous oils. Using some cold and wet cloths can be helpful if you are dealing with swelling and skin irritation.

Edible plants

It is also good to know which plants are considered edible if you need to be able to eat in the wilderness. Keep in mind that you must identify the plant correctly before you are able to eat it. If you look at a plant and are unsure if it is safe or not, it is best to play it safe and not touch it at all. Some of the edible plants that you are able to enjoy in the wilderness include:

Pine trees

Do not confuse the pine tree with other trees. Cedars and cypress will have flattened leaves and firs have short needles. Yews, are poisonous, but also have flat leaves. Pine trees, on the other hand, have long needles and pinecones. Pine needles can be crushed and then used to make a good tea with plenty of vitamin see. Pine nuts are really nutritious and full of the calories and fat that you need to survive.

Berries

There are certain berries that will do well to eat as well, including thimbleberries, raspberries, and blackberries. These are easy to spot and you will be able to collect a ton of them in the late summer to enjoy. Blackberries will be dark purple when they are ripe, but a good raspberry will be completely red. Thimbleberries are a tart relative of the red raspberry and they will be round and bright red when they are ripe. All of these are aggregate berries, so they are safe to eat when you get hungry.

If you have ever grown some of your own strawberries at home, you know that it is easy to tell wild strawberries. They are smaller than the ones that you will find in the store, but they will still be good enough to eat. If you are lucky, your travels may help you to find a large patch of these.

Cattails

If you are in an area that is wet, you will be able to find cattails. The young stems of these are easily eaten raw, but they will taste better when you boil them in water a few minutes. The heads of the flowers are going to be edible in early spring. If the top starts to turn brown and fuzzy, then you should not eat them. You can also peel and cook the roots of the cattail if needed.

Wild grasses and red clover

The flowers, leaves, ands teams of clover can be eaten and then the flowers can be used as a tea. The good thing about this plant is that there are often entire fields of it around to help you stay full. You are able to eat any grass that you want as long as they do not have seeds that are black, pink or purple. This is because they often have a fungus that may kill you. If you have trouble telling what color the seed is, then it is best to not eat it.

You can also choose to eat dandelions. These are small plants that you can find all over the place, which makes them the perfect food to eat. They are recognized by their jagged leaves that will grow right from the ground, as well as their bright yellow flowers. There are some plants that are similar to this, but they do not have the bright yellow flowers. These are fine to eat raw and they will taste like spinach.

There are just a few of the plants that you are able to eat. They may not be your first choice if you were back at home and could go to the grocery store, but if you are really hungry, they are going to do the trick to keep you full and safe when you are lost.

Edible animals

If you spend some time out in the wilderness before you are rescued, you probably do not want to spend all that time eating just plants. There are many animals that you may come across that can be killed, cooked, and then eating. Before you go out and decide to go hunting, there are a few drawbacks that you must consider. If you do decide that it is worth your time to go hunt for food, there are a few animals that will be the best options including:

- Fish: All fish you encounter around you will be edible. Not all of them will taste that great, but they will do if you need sustenance. Sucker fish and some other bottom dwellers will have a muddy taste. Catfish, salmon, bass, and trout will have a much better taste. It is a good idea to carry some fishing supplies in your kit with you to be safe.
- Birds: All birds will be safe to eat as well. So are their eggs. Catching these birds can be an issue though, unless you happen to bring a gun with you. Once you catch the bird, pluck the feathers, skin it, clean it, and then make sure that it is cooked well before you eat.
- Frogs: You are able to eat frogs, but remember that you must leave salamanders and toads alone because most are going to be poisonous. Frog legs are good to eat. You can kill the frogs, skin them, and then cut off the hind legs. Make sure to cook these legs over a fire or boil them.
- Snails, clams, and mussels: If you are near water, there are some sources of food that others will not have. Mussels and claims are

going to be found in bigger bodies of water and they taste good. You should avoid these from the ocean from May to November because these warmer months introduce toxic algae and bacteria that can make these dangerous to eat.
- Snakes: As long as the snake is nonvenomous, they are good to eat. They will be a bit tough to prepare. You need to remove the skin, slice the snake long the belly, and remove the guts in one piece without rupturing them.
- Small mammals: Small animals such as mice, rats, rabbits, and squirrels are edible, but they are hard to catch and they are likely to bite. You need to shoot or trap them and then you have to take the time to skin, clean, and cook them.
- Insects: If you are out in the wilderness long enough, you may need to eat some insects. The best options are large ants, maggots, and grasshoppers. Make sure to cook these up ahead of time because they may contain bacteria and germs, such as tapeworms, that will make you sick.

When you are working with meat, makes sure that you are not cutting your cooked meat with the same knife that you used when you were preparing the meat, at least not without sterilizing it first. You should sterilize the knife after cutting open any raw fish or meat but sticking the blade into the fire or on some hot coals for a minute to help kill anything that might be on the knife and will make you sick.

For the most part, when you get lost in the wilderness, it will only take a short time before people are ready to come look for you and bring you home. This is good news because you will not have to wait around and search for your own food. But with the edible plants and edible meat sources that are listed above, you are sure to find plenty of options that will help keep you safe and full in the wilderness.

Chapter 10: Learning How to Navigate

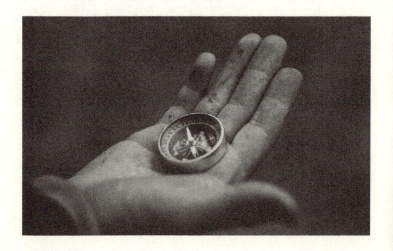

For some people, navigation is an enjoyable puzzle. For others, it is something that is going to lead to a lot of anxiety and will maybe make you more confused and anxious than you were to start with. Being able to properly navigate yourself around when you are lost is the key to helping you get found. It will help you to get back to a main road, or at least get back to where someone is able to find you. There are a few basics that you can start out with to make navigation easier to work with:

- The sun will always rise in the east and set in the west. This can help you to point yourself in the right direction.
- A directional needle on a compass is going to always point to the north. This is how you will be able to use the compass to find your way.
- The easiest way for you to figure out where you are on a map is to place the map in front of you and then look around to see if you find some good landmarks. Is there a road, a lake, a tall mountain? If you find some landmarks, look to see where they are on the map.

All of this will come together to help you to stay safe when you are lost on the trail. Let's look at an example where you are in a campground just south of a big lake. One day you decide to take a friend to go fishing, but you do not have navigation equipment with you. There is a nice trail that circles the entire lake and both of you walk north around the west, or the left, side of the lake for a mile to find your fishing spot.

After being there for a few hours, it is time to head back to camp. But since you do not have a compass, you turn the wrong way, heading north instead of south. You end up walking to the north part of the lake, far away from camp. It is starting to get dark and you are not sure where to go. This is why it is so important to bring along a compass. You would have been able to use it in the scenario above to make sure that you got to the right area on time without getting lost.

Choosing a map

It is also a good idea to choose a map to work with when you are out in the wilderness. There are some types of maps that will be better for those who are exploring the outdoors. A topographic map will show the hills and the mountains that are in the area with a brown and wavy line. The closer the lines get together, the steeper the mountain or hill. And then ever fifth line will show the elevation in feet. With some practice, you will be able to match the outlines that you see on the map to the landmarks that you see around you. These maps will always have north be at the top.

You can also go with an aerial map. These are more like pictures. They are going to show the land around you in the same way that you would be able to see it from an airplane. These are available online easily and you will find that they are helpful in areas that do not have a heavy forest. This is because you will be able to see all the landmarks, such as mountains, buildings, rivers, lakes, and trails in the area. Of course, if you did this in an area that has a lot of forests, all you would be able to see are tree tops. The aerial map will still rely on north being at the top.

If you do not have a map with you, it is possible to make a map as you walk. You can take some paper and draw down all the landmark that you see as you walk by. A mental map will work as well, as long as you are good at noting several landmarks, such as an interesting rock or a fallen tree, as you walk. If you do bring a map, make sure to wrap it in some plastic and seal it up so it does not get wet.

Using your compass

It is important to carry a compass around with you when you are hiking. There are a variety of compass types that you can use, but it is best to go with one that has a mirror and a plastic housing. The mirror is helpful for signaling and the plastic housing will protect the compass. Get in the habit of checking the compass and noting your direction, first as you are exploring, and then periodically as you walk to help you keep on track.

Learning how to read your compass can make a big difference in how safe you stay. The first part of the compass that you need to know about is the directional needle. No matter where you turn, the needle will point to north. The needle is usually red at one end and white or black on the other. The part that is red will be the part that always points north.

This does not mean that the compass is pointing to the North Pole. Instead, compasses are going to point towards a constantly shifting point that is known as the magnetic North Pole. In many places, the distance between the two poles is so great that a compass will need to be adjusted, which can be done by moving a screw or twisting a ring, to help you get a better reading. Your compass should have some instructions on what you can do to adjust it and if you have a topographic map, it will come with a declination number to indicate what adjustments you must make.

Of course, when you are using a compass, you will need to know more directions than just north. While all compass models are different, you should be able to figure out all directions on the compass because the compass housing will have these directions inside. You would be able to turn the compass around to ensure you are going in whatever direction works the best for you.

To read this, you should hold the compass so it is flat in your hand. Turn your body around until you see that the red part of the directional needle is lined up with the orienting arrow. The needle and the orienting arrow need to both be pointing to the north. Once those are set, you will be able to face yourself in the direction that you want to go based on where they are on the compass.

One thing to remember is that to make sure that the compass is working properly, you should keep it away from metal objects, cell phones, and your GPS. This is because the magnetic fields can draw the compass needle in the wrong direction. You should also be careful about extreme conditions that may make the liquid of the compass leak. Keep the hot sun away, insect repellent away, and do not drop your compass.

Other options for orientation

There are times you will be out and you will not have your compass to help you. There are several options you can work with, but never try to determine what direction you are going in based on the belief that moss is only on the north side of a tree or a rock. Moss is able to grow on any side of trees and rocks, especially in a thick forest or a damp area so this is not going to help you that much.

There are several other ways that you will be able to tell which direction you are going in. One way is to use your watch. Hold it with the face up and flat so that it is level with the ground. Then you can line up the hour hand with the sun. next, imagine that there is a line hallway between the hour hand and the 12. This is going to be the north to south line; the part of the line that is ahead of you is south.

If you do not have a watch with you, it is still possible to tell directions. If you know what time it is, you are able to draw a clock in the dirt with the hour hand at the current hour aiming to the sun. then imagine that there is a line halfway between the hour hand and where the 12 of your new clock are. The front part of this line is also going to be pointing to the south.

If you are unsure about what time it is right now, you can choose to make a compass out of a stick and two rocks. Find a spot that is pretty open and then push the stick upright into the ground. Mark where the top of its shadow falls on the rock. Wait about 30 minutes before marking the next shadow with another rock. Stand with the left foot on the first rock and your right foot on the second rock. The direction you are facing is north.

Nighttime is a bit trickier when it comes to telling what direction you are going and if you are in a safe space, it may be best to just stay put. But you can use the stars to help you navigate if needed. Although it seems like the starts move across the sky at night, the polestar, or the North Star, stays pretty close to the same spot, which helps you to figure out where north is. The North Star is easy to find, mainly because it stays put and it is the brightest and biggest star in the sky. The North Star will be the last star in the Little Dipper's hand.

Once you find the North Star, you will be able to place a stick pointing toward it with a rock at one end to mark the north end. When you wake up in the morning, you will then know which direction you should be going. It is best to wait until morning because walking at night can be dangerous since you are not able to see some of the hazards that are around.

GPS

Global Positioning System, or GPS, is another way that you can prevent yourself from getting lost. This is an electronic device that is able to figure out your location by tracking you with satellites. There are several types depending on what you want to use them for, but many have functions like Goto, Compass, and Route. Route is like a map and will show you where you have gone on a map. The Goto function will show you the path to take to get where you want to be, and Compass will place a digital compass on the screen for you.

Every GPS is going to report your location as a set of numbers, and these will be displayed either as standards longitude and latitude numbers, or UTM numbers. With the UTM system, the globe has been flattened and then divided into 60 regions. Your current location will be translated into Eastings and

Northings numbers. It is a good idea to know what number you have so if you communicate with someone, it is easier to find you.

If you plan to go out in the wilderness, it is worth your time to bring along a GPS. They will be able to get a signal almost anywhere you go and they can save a lot of hassle and human error compared to some of the other options that are in this chapter. You will be able to pick where you want to go, whether you would like to use a compass, and even come up with your own coordinates so that you can tell someone else where you are.

Of course, you should be careful with how much you use the GPS and maybe consider having some spare batteries for it if you plan to be gone for a long time. These GPS units usually lose out on power pretty quickly and once it dies out, it will be hard to plug it in while in the wilderness. Also, do not let your GPS or compass be near each other. Each one is going to interfere with the other and that makes it hard to get an accurate reading from either one of them when you need it most.

As you can see, there are several ways that you will be able to tell what direction you are going. It is never a good idea to go out and just wander around and hope that you will be able to get to where you want to go. With these navigational options, you will be able to get out of trouble, and perhaps even get yourself to a location where it is easier for someone to find you.

Chapter 11: Keeping Your Shelter Area Clean

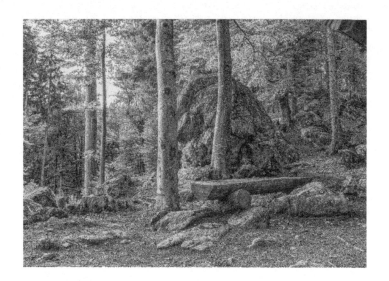

When you are out on the trail and lost, it is important that you not only have a good shelter, but that you also keep it clean. It is not likely that you will be lost for very long since people are searching for you, but even just a few days is enough to attract unwanted company if you do not play it safe. Wild animals will be attracted to the smell of your food and even to your urine so taking care that the area is clean and that things are picked up can help to keep you safe. Let's take a look at some of the things that you can do to ensure that your shelter is clean and that you are able to stay safe.

Food

When it comes to your food, it must be picked up and put away properly. You do not want to attract wild animals because you have left your food out all night for them. This does not mean you can't eat near your shelter, but opening a bag of chips and leaving it wide open is not a good idea either.

The best thing to do is to build your fire a little bit away from your shelter. This helps to keep the likelihood of a fire away from your shelter and moves any smell of the food that you are cooking away as well. That way, if a wild animal is attracted to the food that you are making, they will go near the fire, rather than near you.

Cook and eat your food near the fire as much as possible. And when you are done, do not bring that food back to your shelter or you will still attract the animals. Seal up all the food that is leftover or find a way to dispose of it some distance from your shelter. Leaving it out is just asking for trouble, especially if you bring it back with you. Take the time to clean out your pots and pans and anything else that you used for cooking so that the smell of those doesn't attract the animals either.

If you go out and hunt for your own food, make sure that you store it away from the ground when you are done. Ideally, you only get as much as you are able to eat in one or two sittings so that it doesn't go rotten and doesn't attract some of the animals that you are trying to keep away. For those times when you will need to keep some food and store it, tie up a big strong rope to a tree and store it above the ground. Also, if you do this, make sure that the hanging location is a good distance away from your shelter.

For those who are planning to go out hiking and enjoying the wilderness, consider bringing along some pre-made meals. These are easy to make when you are out in the wilderness and can save you some hassle with finding and preparing the meals that you will eat. They are also easy to store without sending off strong scents to the wild animals when you are not using them.

Making a bathroom

It is also important where you place your bathroom. You do not want to put it right next to the shelter. That is not the most sanitary place to start with and you will end up attracting some wild animals to the area, and that is not good either. Some of the steps that you should take in order to make sure that you are properly handling your waste and going to the bathroom in a way that is sanitary and will keep the wild animals away includes:

- Pick out a spot. You should make sure that this spot is a minimum of 200 feet from your shelter, from the trail, and from any body of water.
- When you find a place, dig a hole. It does not have to be incredibly big, but about six inches deep and eight inches across will do the trick.

- Go to the bathroom.
- Use some wipes if you have them and put them in a baggie. Do not burry this right now because that is hard on the environment and you can throw them away later. As long as they are in the baggie, you will not have to worry about the scent.
- When you are all done, make sure to fill in the whole that you created with soil so that everything is covered up. You want to ensure that the scent is hidden as much as possible so that you do not attract the wild animals.
- Sterilize your hands and make sure that there is nothing left behind when you are done.

And it is simple as that! It does take a little more work compared to just going to the bathroom in the first location you see, but it will help to keep you safe and keep the wild animals away.

Hiding your shelter

The more hidden you can make your shelter, and the more that it matches into the world around you when you are in the wild, the better. When it sticks out or makes a scene, it could attract some unwanted visitors. The good news is that there are several methods that you can use to make sure that your shelter is as hidden as possible. Some of these include:

Build your shelter under the ground.

Building the shelter underground is a good idea if you are able to. This helps to keep the shelter hidden from others and from wild animals, and can also keep you warm and toasty. If the weather is too cold, which makes the ground hard, or there is some other issue, do not worry because the other shelter types can work out well too.

You must be able to find a good place for digging. You want the ground to be nice and sturdy so that the mud will not fall into the shelter on top of you, but it is too hard, you will end up with all the dirt on top of you. It may take a little bit of searching in order to find the perfect spot to dig a hole for your warm shelter area.

Building underground can be worth it, but remember that it does take some time and effort on your part. You must be in good enough shape, physically in terms of your strength and how many injuries you have. When digging the hole, make sure to only dig enough to fit yourself in. Doing more is a waste of your energy and can make it harder to keep the area warm.

Once the shelter is done, make sure to cover up at least the majority of the entry way. Keep a little bit open so that you are able to get some fresh air in while you sleep, but most of it should be closed to protect you and to keep the cold out. A large piece of bark, some leaves, a tarp, or something else that you are able to find around you will do a great job at covering the door and keeping you safe and warm.

Use lots of leaves and pinecones

You may also want to consider using leaves and pinecones to hide your home. There are found in forest and many other places so you should not have to travel too far in order to get the ones that you need. They are free, will not cause any harm to the environment, and will help to keep the shelter warm, no matter which type of shelter you choose to go with.

Try not to leave a mess

No matter how you build your shelter or what type of shelter you choose to go with, it is important that you do not leave a big mess behind. Even if you are using a tarp or some garbage bags, these should not be thrown out when you are done and left to blow around. You should leave the wilderness alone and looking as much the same as it was when you go there as possible.

As you are there, make sure that you look around you after each meal or at least once a day, and consider what you could do to clean up the area. Pick up any paper, wrappers, or anything else that may be lying around. This helps to keep the shelter area looking better and will prevent you from ruining more of the environment than you need to.

When you are rescued, it is still important to look around and clean up. Have someone help you to get the trash bags and tarps off your shelter so those are not left behind if you used them. Clean up anything else that is in the way and that you brought with you.

Keeping your shelter area clean is good for a couple reasons. First, it ensures that you are safe because you are not attracting wild animals to the area from the scents that you leave behind. It can keep you safe because you will not have to worry about tripping over things if you need to use the bathroom in the middle of the night. And it can help to protect the environment and the animals that live there.

Chapter 12: Keeping Dry When it Rains

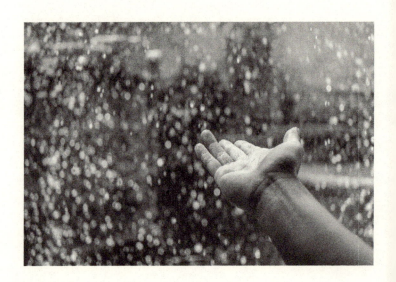

If you are out in the wild for a few days, you will need to deal with rain. Most of the rain that you have will just be a little water and that is it. But sometimes, it is going to include lightning, and this can be dangerous. It is important to be prepared in case it starts to rain.

Even in the case of just a rain shower, you have to be careful. That rain can get on your clothes and may make you cold. If the weather doesn't warm up, you may have some issues with getting chilled and sick. You also have to make sure that your food and other supplies are placed in a shelter, or protected in some other way, so that you can still use them.

In the case of a lightning storm, you have to take extra precautions. You are stuck out in the wild and do not have the regular protection you are used to when you are at home. Staying in a lower area so you are not the tallest thing around, staying away from water, and being in your shelter without any metal will help you to stay safe and sound.

Let's take a look at some of the things that you should to do make sure that you are safe when it is raining, regardless of whether there is lightning that comes along with it.

Get your shelter built and stay in it

If you realize that you are lost when a storm is about to begin, it is time to get that shelter built right away. Staying outside is going to run some risks, such as getting wet and becoming cold or getting struck by lightning if the weather starts to turn bad. The longer you are outside and not in your shelter, the bigger the health risks will become.

If your shelter is not built yet, go to the chapter about making a shelter and get that done as quickly as possible. Digging a shelter underground may be a little hard when the mud is wet and slippery from the rain, but you can use a tarp or other items to help make a different shelter. Go quickly and try to stay away from the tallest trees so you don't attract lightning. Make sure that you do not add any metal or similar options to the shelter, or you risk dealing with electric shock from lightning.

Once the shelter is done, it is best to stay in it until you see that the storm has passed. If you have been lost for some time and the shelter was already built, then go back to the shelter to stay dry. This will ensure that your clothes don't get soaked so you can stay warm and not get sick. It also helps you to avoid being out when lightning comes around.

It is best to stay still and in the shelter until the storm is all gone. It is easy to get lost in a storm when the rain starts to come down fast or when it starts to get dark. This could result in you getting more lost than before. You won't be able to send up many signals, such as a fire signal, while it is raining either. It is much better to stay put during the storm and let others find you. You can do more signaling or looking for food or water when the storm passes.

Stay away from places where lightning strikes

When you are out in the wild and lost, some simple rain showers can turn into big thunderstorms. And when that happens, you may have to deal with lighting. It is important to know how to stay away from lighting so that you do not get electrocuted or harmed from things that are falling over.

The first place you should avoid when you are trying to stay away from lighting is open fields or a hilltop. Lightning is going to strike the tallest object in an area, so do not become that tallest object when you are on a hill or a field. You should pick a lower area, like a ravine or a valley, and try to stay away from the rain as much as possible. Stay there, crouching down with the heels to the ground and your head between your knees if you are stuck out in the weather because this helps to make you a smaller target. You do not want to lie flat on the ground though because lighting has the potential to be fatal up to a hundred feet from where it strikes.

Stay out of the water when it is raining. If you are already in the water when the thunderstorm starts, it is time to get to land right away. Once you are out, it is important that you do not get back into that water for at least thirty minutes after the last lightning strike you saw. If you go in earlier, the storm may still be going on and you can get hurt.

When you are looking for shelter, if you do not have one created already, do not stand near a tall isolated object or trees. These taller objects are more likely to be struck with lightning. No matter where you are, it is important to avoid standing under a tree in a lightning storm and make sure you stay away from any tall objects, like light posts. If you are in the forest, you should stay near a lower stand of trees. It is also a good idea to put the umbrella away when you start to see the lightning.

You should also try to avoid metal objects, like fences or pipes that are exposed if you see any that are near you. Metal is going to conduct electricity, and this makes it more likely that you will get hit if lightning strikes. If you have some metal objects on you, let them go until after the storm has passed. If you have an electronic device, such as a GPS or some piercings, these are not really large enough to cause an issue so it is fine to hold onto them.

If you happen to have something like a bike on you during this time, then it is best to drop the bike and then crouch down to the ground if there is lightning nearby. Most good bikes are going to be made out of metal and they are excellent lightning conductors so it is best to stay away from them. Rubber objects, like your rubber shoes, are not going to be able to protect you from the conducting properties that come with metal, whether we are talking about your bike or something else.

Wear the right clothing

If you are lost on the trail, it is likely going to rain. This just seems to be the way that things go. So, if you plan on being out on the trail at all, it is probably a good idea to make sure that you are wearing the right clothing. This is going to be similar to what we talked about with winter and getting stuck in the cold, but there are a few differences when it comes to rain.

You should make sure that the jacket you are wearing is waterproof as well as breathable. The waterproof means that when it rains, the water will stay off you and will not cause you to get cold or sick in the process. The breathable is important because if you sweat a lot, it will ensure that the sweat does not stick to you at all. Also, the jacket should have a hood and a zip that you can open and shut for some ventilation.

The right clothes are also important. You should stay away from cotton if it is going to rain, whether it is cold or warm. Cotton may help to keep you cooler, but no one wants to have all that rain collect on a cotton shirt and then just stay their forever. Cotton is known for collecting water, whether it is snow, rain, or sweat, and then will hold it close to your body. If it is a warm day, this may not be so bad, but if it is cool at all, this could make you feel pretty miserable.

Some waterproof and breathable pants can be a nice addition as well. These will make it easier to walk around if the weather gets rainy and will not drag you down if the rain starts to come.

A good hat and an umbrella may be nice if it is going to rain quite a bit. A polyester or nylon baseball cap will help to keep the water out of your eyes while you are walking. If you plan to be out in the rain at all when you are hiking, consider bringing that cap along to help you stay safe.

Underneath the rain gear, wear some wool or synthetic base layer, like a lightweight long underwear or some running tights and a tech tee. If you are not able to wear some waterproof pants, these end up getting really hot, which can be hard in summer, it is best to go with something that is water-resistant. If you were able to plan ahead of time before going out, you should keep a warm layer, such as a fleece jacket in your pack to help you out if it gets cold. The most important thing to remember is that you need to avoid cotton clothing because it will soak up all that water when it rains and it is not able to keep you warm when it rains.

Some waterproof hiking boots can be a good idea as well and they will make you so much more comfortable when you are on soggy trails. The boots will help to provide some extra traction that you need to not fall over while you are walking. They are also heavy duty enough that you are able to keep your feet dry, even if you are out in the rain.

Avoiding flash floods

Most of the time, when you encounter rain, it will just be a little storm and then it is all over. But occasionally, depending on the time of year and where you get lost, you may have to deal with a flash flood. A flash flood is going to start with unusually hard rains, such as four inches or more in an hour, or when there is a substantial amount of rain for a few days in a row. In areas that are arid and hot, the sun can bake the dirt so much that this soil is not able to soak up the water at all. When this happens, the water will run down the walls of a canyon and will start a smallish creek at the bottom. It will not take long before this turns into a raging river.

If the rain is strong for a few days, the canyons and creek beds are going to become saturated and they will not be able to hold onto any more water. The same thing as above is going to occur. The dry creek beds will keep on filling, and then fast flowing rivers will flow.

If you are hiking in certain areas, you probably already know whether you would be affected by a flood. Canyons are big areas where these occur, as can dry creek beds. If you are near these areas, you must be careful. For example, staying out of a canyon and not building your shelter too close to a river or creek, especially when it is going to rain, can help to save your life.

There are some warning signs that show up when a flash flood is about to happen. If you are in a canyon or another place that is a candidate for flash flooding and you hear some thunder, it is time to get out. If you start to feel a stiff breeze in the canyon towards you or there is a roaring sound, it is time to think quick because the flash flood is already heading your way.

When you get to this point, it is time to look for higher ground, or at least a way that you can get out of the situation. While you are hiking, always look for a way that you can get out just in case. Are there ways that you are able to scramble out of the canyon if you need, for example. Knowing these escape routes ahead of time will be beneficial when you start to hear a flash flood coming your way. It prevents you from having to waste time panicking and looking around. You will simply need to start heading for the exit you saw and you are then set to get out safe.

If you are planning on going out on a hike and you hear that the weather reports are talking about substantial amounts of rain in the area you would like to hike in, then it is best to pick another place to hike or to wait for another day. It is much better to stay safe rather than get caught in a flash flood. In the desert, it is possible that big amounts of rain that occur 100 mils away could potentially cause flash floods where you are going. If you know that there are some big storms in the area or that it is monsoon season, it is best to play it safe and go hiking on higher ground.

Staying safe when it rains is so important. You want to make sure that you are taking care of yourself and that you do not get too wet or cold along the way. You should only be lost on the trail for a few days at most, but one cold rain could make you really sick and could turn the situation worse. But if you are able to stay out of the rain or wear the right clothes when you are in the rain, it will make life easier until you can be found.

Chapter 13: How to Survive Extreme Weather

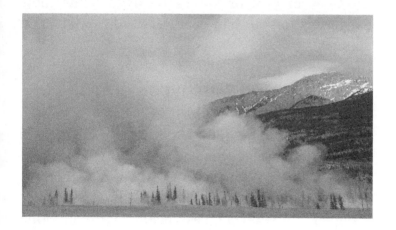

When you think about dangers in the wilderness that would harm or kill you, it is likely that the first thing that you will think about includes rattlesnakes, lions, and bears. However, one of the biggest threats that will happen to you from being lost in the wilderness will include falling, drowning, and extreme weather. Without putting together the proper shelter and without the right supplies, extremes in cold or hot can end up being more dangerous to you than dealing with bears or other animals.

Dealing with hypothermia

If you are out in weather that is cold, or any time in the winter when the temperatures can drop down quickly, you may have to worry about hypothermia. Hypothermia means that your body temperature dropped a few degrees below normal. Mild hypothermia is something that you can fix without too much trouble, but severe hypothermia, especially if it last a long time, will be deadly.

So, how do you become hypothermic? There are several ways that you will lose body heat. Resting or sitting on cold ground can pull out body heat. Sweating from exercise when it is cold out can also make your body cool down too quickly. If you breathe in the cold air too quickly or you are out exposed to the cold wind, you will cool down quickly.

The first signs that you will notice with hypothermia are going to be shivering and goose bumps. Shivering is a sign that your body is trying to create more heat because it is moving your muscles. You may start out with just a little shivering, but as the body gets colder, it is possible that you will start to shake all over. Your skin can turn red, just like it was sunburnt. You may find that you are not able to easily touch your thumb and your little finger.

A good sign that you are dealing with hypothermia is that you are dealing with the umbles: the fumbles, mumbles, stumbles, and tumbles. This means that you are starting to get clumsy, you experience some issues with speaking, will becomes confused, and completing tasks is hard. You may not have energy, feel sleepy, and start to think that it is not important what happens to you because you just want to be left alone. The issue of hypothermia will keep going until your heart rate starts to slow down. You may even feel warm for a bit, even tough you are not.

There are a few things that you can do to help keep yourself warm when you are out in the cold and will ensure that you are not going to catch hypothermia including:

- Wear a lot of clothing: It is a good idea to wear two to three layers of clothing when you go out in the cold. These clothes should be loose fitting so that the air will be able to get through and keep you warm compared to wearing just one layer.
- Avoid any cotton clothing: Cotton may be comfortable, but it will get wet when it is cold, if you wear cotton when it is raining or snowing, you will lose a lot of heat out of your body and it will not take long for your body to chill. Polyester and fleece clothing will hold in the body heat and insulates it from the cold.
- Keep your hands, neck, and head covered up. This is a simple idea, but it is one that a lot of people will forget about. You are going to lose a lot of your body heat from the neck and head. A fleece hat does not take up much room in your bag, but it can be enough to save your life. And always carry around a

pair of mittens or gloves to keep your hands warm.

- Always stay dry: Damp clothing is going to make your body really cold. If you are out in wet weather and you are not wearing waterproof clothing at the top layer, you should cover yourself up with some trash bags to help stay dry. You can also use smaller bags on the hands to keep dry. If you do happen to get wet, make sure that you build up a fire as quickly as possible to warm up yourself and your clothes.
- Never wear clothing that overheats you: Clothes that make you sweat will absorb that sweat and then become damp. If you have to haul wood or build a shelter and it is cold, you should take of your outer layer of clothing (or your coat), so that you do not sweat as much. You can put it back on later when you are all done.
- Stay protected from the wind: Windchill is a term that will describe how cold the temperature feels to animals and people when the cooling effects of that wind are taken into account. Wind will pull the heat off your body. This is why you are going to feel so much cooler on days when it is cold and windy compared to days that are just

cold. Find some shelter to stay out of the wind to help keep yourself warm.

- Eat foods that have a lot of calories: Calories will give you energy and energy will help you to keep warm. Take along some easy to carry high calorie foods like almonds, peanuts, and chocolate to help you out.
- Stay active: The more active you can be, the easier it is to stay warm when it is cold. Do jumping jacks, run in place, and move around to get the blood to circulate around. While you are doing this, you should take off a few layers of clothing while you are doing this so that you do not sweat at the same time. Put the clothing back on when you are done.
- Find ways to insulate: If you start to feel cold, stuff your clothing with some pine needles, dry leaves, or something else that will keep the body safe from the wind and cold temperatures. A layer of just leaves between the jacket and your shirt can help to keep you warm. A trash bag as your outer layer and then some grass in there will work as well.
- Drink enough fluids: When you feel dehydrated, you will find that your blood will not flow as well and this makes you feel cold so much faster. You can help to keep the

body warm with plenty of water. Warm water is best, but if all you have is cold, it is better than nothing. Add some sugar to the water to help give you a boost in calories as well.
- Stay by the fire: If you were able to get a fire going, then you should stay by this until it warms up. This will make it easier to keep your body warm so you do not become hypothermic.

If you start to feel hypothermic, you should slowly heat your body up. If you try to bring up the temperature too quickly, it is going to be a shock to the system. Start by sitting by your fire with a blanket, then add on some heat packets, and so on so that your body has time to slowly warm up.

Frostbite

In the cold weather, it is also possible that you may deal with frostbite in the skin and other tissues because a particular part of your body is starting to freeze. It is possible to have severe and mild forms of frostbite depending on how frozen that body parts become. The most likely places to get frostbite include on your face, nose, ears, hands, and feet. Some of the signs that you are dealing with frostbite include:

- A part of your skin starts to look white or grayish.
- If you get a feeling like pins and needs followed by numbness
- The area is aching or throbbing with pain.
- The area feels like it is a block of wood. This means that you are not able to feel anything there and the flesh looks hard and pale.

As soon as you start to notice any of these signs when it comes to hypothermia, it is time to warm up and move that area of the body. Wriggle around your toes and clench your fists. Make funny faces, scrunch it around and do what you can to warm it up. Take your hands from the mittens and use them to warm your nose or ears. If your fingers start to hurt, tuck the hands into the jacket and under your armpits to help warm them up. Do anything that you can to help keep the area warm.

Once you have developed frostbite that is severe, the worst thing that you are going to do is try to thaw that skin, have it freeze again and then rewarm it. What this means for you if you are stuck in the wild is that unless you are sure that you can get over to a hospital right away, or unless you are sure that you can keep that area dry and warm until you are rescued, it is not a good idea to warm or thaw the areas of your body that are really frostbitten.

Heat illness

There will be times when you get lost out in the heat as well. It is important to drink plenty of water and protect yourself from the sun, or you can get just as sick as you can with the cold. Heat exhaustion can be a mildly uncomfortable issue, but it is possible for it to turn into a fatal condition that is known as heat stroke. The symptoms that you should watch out for when dealing with heat exhaustion include:

- Cool and damp skin
- Dark urine or not being able to go pee
- Muscle cramps
- Headaches
- Fever
- Heavy sweating
- Fainting
- Feeling sick to your stomach or dizzy
- Tired and weak

If you are dealing with any of these symptoms, it is time to get your body cooled down right away. Get in the shade and if you are able to, get to some cool water. Drink as much water as you can, even if you do not feel that thirsty at the time. If you are wearing clothes that are tight or heavy, it is time to loosen them up and even remove them. If you are able to wet the clothes that you are wearing, then this is the time to do it. Since the ground is going to be cooler under the surface, it is a good idea to dig down a bit if you have the energy.

For those who plan to be out in the heat, it is best to wear lightweight clothing so that you can keep the sun off your skin but not get too hot from the clothing. Unlike with cold weather, cotton clothing can be the best for hot weather because it will keep you cool. Wearing a hot, especially one with a net around it to keep bugs off, can help you to stay cool in the hot sun. some people bring along a bandana because you can wet this and tie it around your neck to keep cool, and they also work as a hat if needed.

Snow or sun blindness

When you are staring at UV rays from the sun for hours, it could cause a sunburn on your corneas. People will blue or green eyes are going to be the most susceptible to this, but anyone who is around a surface that is highly reflective, such as desert sand or snow, is at risk. Burning your corneas can hurt. It will feel like a scratch is in your eye, such as when there is dust in it. After some time, you will feel some sharp pain and it will be hard to open your eyes. If the case gets severe, your eyes may become damaged and it is possible to go blind temporarily.

To make sure that you do not end up with eye damage to start with, wear some sunglasses, use a hat to shade your eyes, or tie some cloth on your eyes like a blindfold with a small slit for you to look from. You can also make some eyeshades with the help of plastic or bark so that less light is going to hit your eyes.

How to deal with mudslides

Another issue you may encounter when you are out on the trail are mudslides. A mudslide will occur when there is a lot of water and an area of loose soil that this water is able to soak into. If the area of soil is on a hill, then there is not much that will keep it from going down. This can then turn into a mudslide, with trees, boulders, and other things in the way going down with it.

The lack of any stabilizing feature is a big component of a mudslide forming. The roots from plants, grass, and trees will do a lot to stabilize the ground and will stop erosion. When these are not around, there is not much to stop a mudslide from happening. If you are hiking in an area that is on a side of a hill or a mountain and there isn't much vegetation, you are in the prime location for a mudslide to occur.

There are a few things that you can do to make sure that you are safe and aware when it comes to dealing with a mudslide. First, you must be aware of what is going on around you to avoid being caught right in the middle of a mudslide. You should know when you are in an area where a mudslide is likely to happen and you should be aware of the weather that is going on there. Remember that to get a mudslide to form, you need massive amounts of water, such as from a rainstorm or even when snow is melting quickly in the spring.

You also want to get as high up as possible when a mudslide occurs. These mudslides are going to go quick and they will bring a lot of material with them, such as trees, rocks, and anything else that is found on the hill. If you are down low, you may get hit with these and not be able to do anything about it. Being on higher ground can keep you safe.

Mudslides are able to move really quickly, similar to an avalanche. There is no real way that you are able to outrun it. If you are already outside when it happens, the best thing to do is find a shelter or getting up as high as possible. If you must run because there are no other options, then you should get out of the way from the mudslide and then run crosswise so you are going across the face of the mountainside. This is going to help you to move yourself out of the way of the mud and it is a lot faster than running downhill and trying to race it.

Working with forest fires

Depending on the time of year that you get lost and your location, you may need to deal with forest fires. A forest fire can sometimes be small, but it can grow to be huge and hard to control depending on what is going on around you. Sometimes these forest fires are going to be started by nature, but there are times when they are started by humans. Sometimes they are started on purpose, and other times they are started on accident.

Forest fires that are started by nature are often started by lightning, though there are some times when a hot sun in an arid area will cause a fire. Once these fires start, it is hard to stop them. They usually start far away from others and since no one sees them getting started, they can quickly grow big and take over before anyone even notices.

Humans can also start fires, whether it is intentional or not. You could start a fire as a signal to help people to find you, or to cook food and stay warm, but if you do not take the proper care of it or if you do not fully get it to stop burning, you could start a forest fire. Other times, someone may decide to perform arson and will get the area to burn.

You do not want to be out when it comes to a forest fire. The first thing that you should do when you are planning on going on a hike is to check if the area you will hike in is prone to a forest fire while you are there. In an area that is managed, there will be signs to let you know if there is danger for a wildfire. It is important to remember that even if a fire is not common in that area, you should still be on the look-out. If you go to an area that has a long drought period and a storm is about to start, you could be in a risk area.

If a forest fire starts, it is important to stay calm and think through things. Some of the tips that you can follow to make sure that you stay safe when there is a forest fire includes:

- Get out of that area: If you are able to get away from the fire, move as quickly as you safely can away. You should also figure out which direction the wind is going if possible. This will help you to know whether the fire will follow you or will go the other way. If you are not able to get away, look for a shelter that will be able to help protect you until the fire is gone.
- If there is some kind of fire break that occurs near you, such as a road or a river, cross over to the other side. You can look on your map to see if one of these are nearby to keep you safe.
- If you get caught in an oncoming forest, you should move over to an area where no vegetation is present. This means that the fire will not be able to grow in that area. A rocky area or a lake are good options. The bigger the area is, the better because it will keep the fire away and will help you to not inhale the fire smoke.
- Never go down into a valley if the fire is already burning there. It is always better to leave as many ridges between the fire and you as possible because this can provide some defense to you.
- If a forest fire was just done, you should be careful walking through an area that has

smoldering vegetation or burnt ground. Burning branches will fall from trees or there could be fire flashes on the ground that could harm you.
- If you are in the fire and there doesn't seem to be a way to get out, then it is time to find the barest patch of ground that you can. The less vegetation there is to burn, the better. Lie down on it with your face down and do your best to cover yourself with the surrounding soil. This will give you some air filtering and the soil on your clothes and body will hopefully help you to stay protected.

If you have the ability to plan the hike ahead of time, it is best to avoid going into areas that are known to have forest fires. These can be scary to deal with and you never know for sure which way a fire will go. If you do get stuck in a forest fire, keep your wits about you and try to keep as much distance between yourself and the fire, even if you have to go off the path a bit, to ensure you can stay safe until it passes.

There are all sorts of bad weather out there that you may have to deal with. It all depends on when you get out in the open what you will need to deal with. Make sure that when you go out, you have a good idea of how the weather will behave, and keep a few things on you to keep yourself protected.

Principles of surviving extreme weather

There are a lot of different kinds of extreme weather that you may encounter when it comes to being left alone in the wilderness. The best thing that you can do is be prepared. Even if the weather has been nice in the area and there are no imminent threats around, it is still a good idea to plan for the worst. By following these basic principles, you will be able to get through, no matter what the weather throws at you.

Always be prepared when you leave home

Before you go out, whether you are on a road trip, going to the town nearby, or heading out on the trail, it is always a good idea to be prepared. Err on the side of caution if you can because you never know when things are not going to turn out the way that you plan. Having some comfortable clothes that match the current weather, plenty of water, some food, and a first aid kit can go a long way to ensuring that you are able to survive until you are fine, no matter what kind of weather you meet.

Look at the forecast

While the forecast seems to be inaccurate at times, it will be able to help you get a general idea of what to expect. If there is a warning about a severe storm coming up, it is probably not a good idea to go out and hike at this time. If it is going to be record highs, you should bring along some sunscreen and some extra water or stay at home.

You can also take a look at some of the records of what has happened in the area you are traveling at this time of year. The weatherman may not tell the whole story sometimes and looking back at the history of the weather in that area could tell you a lot about what you can expect.

Be boring and conservative

While it may not bring out as big of a tail or be as interesting, when you are out in the wilderness, especially if you are dealing with some extremes in weather, it is best to just keep it boring. You should simply stay where you are, don't take any risks that you do not need to do, and wait for someone to come and find you. This may not make the most interesting television show, but it is the best way to survive and get found quickly, without getting in harms way.

If you have food and water on you, and it is extremely hot or blizzarding out, do not go out. You can even go a few days without food if needed and if you do not move around a lot, your water supply will last you some time. In the heat, only move when needed to keep get water and the necessities. In the cold, take some snow and warm it up so that you don't become dehydrated. Otherwise, just stay in one spot. Moving around too much puts you at risk of getting lost or harmed, and it is much safer to stay put until someone else is able to find you.

Use your common sense

When you are lost on the trail, it is important to use your common sense as much as possible. This can be hard when you are scared and tired and alone, but it really will help you. For example, there are a ton of people who choose to drive across a flooded roadway, even though they know they shouldn't, because they get anxious and worried in the moment. Many people will stay around water when there is a lightning storm for the same reason. You know that you should go up to a higher point around you and then try your cell phone or GPS if it is not working. But when you are lost and scared you are not thinking straight, and these common sense ideas seem to go out the window.

If you are struggling to figure out what you need to get done, then it is time to take a break and relax. It is normal to feel worked up and anxious when you first get lost, but letting these emotions get in the mix will just lead you to more mistakes. It is better to take a step back and stop whatever you are doing than it is to keep going and make mistakes that can put you in harms way or will make it harder for people to find you later.

Conclusion

Thank for making it through to the end of this book, let's hope it was informative and able to provide you with all of the tools you need to achieve your goals whatever they may be.

The next step is to make sure that you understand all the steps that you should take to stay safe if you need to survive in the wilderness. The more that you know these skills, the less scary it can be to stay out there until someone is able to find you. The worst thing that you can do for yourself when you are lost is to get nervous and upset, even though those are normal reactions to the situation, and being prepared will help you to stay calm.

This guidebook spent some time looking at the different things that you must take care of when you are surviving in the wilderness. We looked at how to get water, how to build a good shelter, ways to avoid wild animals, which foods you are able to eat, and even how to survive in extreme weather conditions. There are so many things that you will need to do when you get stuck in the wilderness, and all the topics in this guidebook will help you to get there.

When you are ready to start learning some new survival skills and you want to make sure you are prepared in cause you ever do get lost in the wilderness, make sure to read through this guidebook to get the answers you need.

Finally, if you found this book useful in anyway, a review on Amazon is always appreciated! Send your critics and suggestion to <u>support@weiseweasel.com</u>

Made in the USA
Las Vegas, NV
29 May 2021